NATIONAL ACADEMIES

Sciences
Engineering
Medicine

NATIONAL
ACADEMIES
PRESS
Washington, DC

T0073582

Using Population Descriptors in Genetics and Genomics Research

A New Framework for an Evolving Field

Committee on the Use of Race, Ethnicity, and Ancestry
as Population Descriptors in Genomics Research

Board on Health Sciences Policy

Health and Medicine Division

Committee on Population

Division of Behavioral and Social Sciences and Education

Consensus Study Report

NATIONAL ACADEMIES PRESS 500 Fifth Street, NW, Washington, DC 20001

This project has been funded with federal funds under Contract No. HHSN263201800029I (75N98021F00009) between the National Academy of Sciences and the Department of Health and Human Services, National Institutes of Health: All of Us Research Program; National Cancer Institute; National Heart, Lung, and Blood Institute; National Human Genome Research Institute; Eunice Kennedy Shriver National Institute of Child Health and Human Development; National Institute of Dental and Craniofacial Research; National Institute of Diabetes and Digestive and Kidney Diseases; National Institute of Environmental Health Sciences; National Institute of Nursing Research; National Institute on Aging; National Institute on Drug Abuse; National Institute on Minority Health and Health Disparities; NIH Office of Behavioral and Social Sciences Research; and NIH Office of Science Policy. Any opinions, findings, conclusions, or recommendations expressed in this publication do not necessarily reflect the views of any organization or agency that provided support for the project.

International Standard Book Number-13: 978-0-309-70065-8
International Standard Book Number-10: 0-309-70065-5
Digital Object Identifier: https://doi.org/10.17226/26902

This publication is available from the National Academies Press, 500 Fifth Street, NW, Keck 360, Washington, DC 20001; (800) 624-6242 or (202) 334-3313; http://www.nap.edu.

Suggested citation: National Academies of Sciences, Engineering, and Medicine. 2023. *Using population descriptors in genetics and genomics research: A new framework for an evolving field.* Washington, DC: The National Academies Press. https://doi.org/10.17226/26902.

The **National Academy of Sciences** was established in 1863 by an Act of Congress, signed by President Lincoln, as a private, nongovernmental institution to advise the nation on issues related to science and technology. Members are elected by their peers for outstanding contributions to research. Dr. Marcia McNutt is president.

The **National Academy of Engineering** was established in 1964 under the charter of the National Academy of Sciences to bring the practices of engineering to advising the nation. Members are elected by their peers for extraordinary contributions to engineering. Dr. John L. Anderson is president.

The **National Academy of Medicine** (formerly the Institute of Medicine) was established in 1970 under the charter of the National Academy of Sciences to advise the nation on medical and health issues. Members are elected by their peers for distinguished contributions to medicine and health. Dr. Victor J. Dzau is president.

The three Academies work together as the **National Academies of Sciences, Engineering, and Medicine** to provide independent, objective analysis and advice to the nation and conduct other activities to solve complex problems and inform public policy decisions. The National Academies also encourage education and research, recognize outstanding contributions to knowledge, and increase public understanding in matters of science, engineering, and medicine.

Learn more about the National Academies of Sciences, Engineering, and Medicine at **www.nationalacademies.org**.

Consensus Study Reports published by the National Academies of Sciences, Engineering, and Medicine document the evidence-based consensus on the study's statement of task by an authoring committee of experts. Reports typically include findings, conclusions, and recommendations based on information gathered by the committee and the committee's deliberations. Each report has been subjected to a rigorous and independent peer-review process, and it represents the position of the National Academies on the statement of task.

Proceedings published by the National Academies of Sciences, Engineering, and Medicine chronicle the presentations and discussions at a workshop, symposium, or other event convened by the National Academies. The statements and opinions contained in proceedings are those of the participants and are not endorsed by other participants, the planning committee, or the National Academies.

Rapid Expert Consultations published by the National Academies of Sciences, Engineering, and Medicine are authored by subject-matter experts on narrowly focused topics that can be supported by a body of evidence. The discussions contained in rapid expert consultations are considered those of the authors and do not contain policy recommendations. Rapid expert consultations are reviewed by the institution before release.

For information about other products and activities of the National Academies, please visit www.nationalacademies.org/about/whatwedo.

---

[1] See Appendix F, Disclosure of Unavoidable Conflict of Interest.

ANDRÉS MORENO-ESTRADA, Professor, Advanced Genomics Unit, Centro de Investigación y de Estudios Avanzados del Instituto Politécnico Nacional (CINVESTAV), Mexico

ANN MORNING, James Weldon Johnson Professor of Sociology, New York University

JOHN P. NOVEMBRE, Professor, Department of Human Genetics, Department of Ecology & Evolution, University of Chicago

MOLLY PRZEWORSKI, Professor, Department of Biological Sciences, Department of Systems Biology, Columbia University

DOROTHY E. ROBERTS, George A. Weiss University Professor of Law & Sociology; Raymond Pace & Sadie Tanner Mossell Alexander Professor of Civil Rights; Professor of Africana Studies; Director, Penn Program on Race, Science & Society, University of Pennsylvania

SARAH A. TISHKOFF, David and Lyn Silfen University Professor, Departments of Genetics and Biology; Director, Center for Global Genomics & Health Equity, University of Pennsylvania

GENEVIEVE L. WOJCIK, Assistant Professor of Epidemiology, Department of Epidemiology, Johns Hopkins Bloomberg School of Public Health

Study Staff

SARAH H. BEACHY, Study Director

SAMANTHA N. SCHUMM, Associate Program Officer

LEAH CAIRNS, Study Codirector *(until October 2022)*

KATHRYN ASALONE, Associate Program Officer

MEREDITH HACKMANN, Associate Program Officer

LYDIA TEFERRA, Research Assistant

APARNA CHERAN, Senior Program Assistant *(from June 2022)*

MICHAEL K. ZIERLER, Science Writer

ANDREW M. POPE, Senior Director, Board on Health and Sciences Policy *(until July 2022)*

CLARE STROUD, Senior Director, Board on Health and Sciences Policy *(from July 2022)*

MALAY K. MAJMUNDAR, Director, Committee on Population

Reviewers

This Consensus Study Report was reviewed in draft form by individuals chosen for their diverse perspectives and technical expertise. The purpose of this independent review is to provide candid and critical comments that will assist the National Academies of Sciences, Engineering, and Medicine in making each published report as sound as possible and to ensure that it meets the institutional standards for quality, objectivity, evidence, and responsiveness to the study charge. The review comments and draft manuscript remain confidential to protect the integrity of the deliberative process.

We thank the following individuals for their review of this report:

WENDY CHUNG, Columbia University
DANA A. GLEI, Georgetown University
EVELYNN M. HAMMONDS, Harvard University
CHANITA HUGHES-HALBERT, University of Southern California
BENJAMIN NEALE, Harvard Medical School
NEIL R. POWE, University of California, San Francisco
ERICA RAMOS, Genome Medical
ALIYA SAPERSTEIN, Stanford University
THE REVEREND ROBERT JEMONDE TAYLOR, Duke Cancer
     Institute Community Advisory Council
SHARON F. TERRY, Genetic Alliance
HONGYU ZHAO, Yale University

Although the reviewers listed above provided many constructive comments and suggestions, they were not asked to endorse the conclusions or recommendations of this report nor did they see the final draft before its release. The review of this report was overseen by **SUSAN J. CURRY** of the University of Iowa and **LINDA C. DEGUTIS** of the Yale School of Public Health. They were responsible for making certain that an independent examination of this report was carried out in accordance with the standards of the National Academies and that all review comments were carefully considered. Responsibility for the final content rests entirely with the authoring committee and the National Academies.

Acknowledgments

The study committee and project staff acknowledge that the National Academies of Sciences, Engineering, and Medicine is physically housed on the traditional land of the Nacotchtank (Anacostan) and Piscataway Peoples, past and present. The committee and staff honor with gratitude the land itself and the people who have stewarded it throughout the generations. They honor and respect the enduring relationship that exists between these peoples and nations and this land. The committee and staff thank these peoples for their resilience in protecting this land and aspire to uphold our responsibilities to their example. The committee and staff also acknowledge the countless number of people who have participated, both willingly and unwillingly, in biomedical research, as well as those who have raised the issues addressed in this study for many years.

The study committee and project staff would like to thank the study sponsor—the 14 institutes, program, and offices of the National Institutes of Health—for their leadership on this issue and for their vision and commitment to developing and supporting this project. The committee and staff express their gratitude to the many experts who shared their diverse perspectives and advice with the committee throughout the process and during the public sessions. The committee is grateful for the staff within the Health and Medicine Division who provided support and guidance for the project, along with their collaborators in the Division of Behavioral and Social Sciences and Education.

Contents

6 IMPLEMENTATION AND ACCOUNTABILITY   149

Introduction, 149
Implementation Across the Genomics Research Ecosystem, 150
Recommendations, 159
Mechanisms of Accountability, 160
Parting Thoughts, 161
References, 162

APPENDIXES

List of Boxes, Figures, and Tables

BOXES

FIGURES

TABLES

Preface

Human genetics studies that assess the contributions of genes to phenotypes can be conducted either using relatives or groups of distantly related individuals ("unrelated" in a colloquial sense). In both instances, geneticists search for a pattern of genetic (sequence or allelic) variation that can distinguish between different forms of a phenotype, say, individuals with sickle cell anemia from those with sickle cell trait, based on the known rules of Mendelian genetic transmission. Although the expected similarity or dissimilarity of closely related individuals largely depends on gene transmission rules, that between more distantly related individuals mostly depends on their remote ancestral histories, such as where, when, and how their common ancestors arose. This information is partially captured by affiliation of an individual to a population; however, how a population should be defined for any specific question in genetics research is less clear. Nevertheless, for any human genetics research, now extended to entire genomes, it is critical to clearly describe who is selected for a study, why, and how. Researchers also need to specify the criteria used to describe participants, including the use of population descriptors. Unfortunately, genetics studies have not named individuals consistently or in a principled manner, often reflexively using race and ethnicity without great thought or justification. Though seldom studied, measures of the environments associated with study individuals and groups are also germane to our understanding of genetic traits and disorders and need to be included.

In recent years, genetic information has become far more accessible. The number of human genetics and genomics studies is rapidly increasing, and many such studies are led by investigators who were not primarily trained in human genetics. While this study focuses mainly on knowledge from human genetics and genomics, we acknowledge that knowledge from many other sources (oral, archaeological, traditional, community, etc.) serves to inform our identities, history, relationships to other humans, and our traits and diseases. *It is time for us to reshape how genetics studies are conceptualized, conducted, and interpreted.*

This commissioned study describes an effort to clarify the scientific rationales for describing research participants and their group labels. We start with a historical view of how we got to our current state, then proceed to examine how else we could achieve our scientific aims, and follow with our recommendations and suggested implementations to improve genetic and genomic science. Our overarching goal is to motivate researchers to consider when population descriptors are necessary, which ones are appropriate for a specific type of genetics study design, whether multiple descriptors are necessary, and what additional information is needed for genetic dissection of phenotypes. Accordingly, this report is divided into two sections; the first is "Past and Current Use of Population Descriptors," and the second section is "Recommendations."

Aravinda Chakravarti and Charmaine Royal,
Cochairs, Committee on the Use of Race, Ethnicity, and
Ancestry as Population Descriptors in Genomics Research

Abbreviations

1000G	1000 Genomes Project; the international 1000 genomes sequence variation project
AAA	American Anthropological Association
AAPA	American Association of Physical Anthropologists
AFR	African "superpopulation"
AMA	American Medical Association
APA	American Psychological Association
APOE4	apolipoprotein E gene
BBJ	BioBank Japan
BIPMed	Brazilian Initiative on Precision Medicine
CDC	Centers for Disease Control and Prevention
CDE	common data element
CEPH	northern and western European ancestry in Utah
CEU	northern European in Utah
CKB	China Kadoorie Biobank
CONSORT	Consolidated Standards of Reporting Trials
COREQ	COnsolidated criteria for REporting Qualitative research
COVID-19	coronavirus disease 2019
DNA	deoxyribonucleic acid
EUR	European "superpopulation"

FAPESP	Research Innovation and Dissemination Centers funded by the São Paulo Research Foundation
GBR	British in England and Scotland
GIH	Gujaratis sampled in Houston
gnomAD	Genome Aggregation Database
GWAS	genome-wide association study
HAALSI	Health and Aging in Africa: A Longitudinal Study of an INDEPTH Community in South Africa
HAAO	3-hydroxyanthranilate 3,4-dioxygenase
HapMap	International Haplotype Map Project
HGP	Human Genome Project
HIV	human immunodeficiency virus
HLA	human leukocyte antigen
HMD	Health and Medicine Division
INDEPTH	International Network for the Demographic Evaluation of Populations and Their Health
JAMA	*Journal of the American Medical Association*
KBP	Korean Biobank Project
KYNU	kynureninase
LD	linkage disequilibrium
MeSH	Medical Subject Headings
mRNA	messenger RNA
MXB	Mexican Biobank
NAD	nicotinamide adenine dinucleotide
NHGRI	National Human Genome Research Institute
NHLBI	National Heart, Lung, and Blood Institute
NIH	National Institutes of Health
NIMHD	National Institute on Minority Health and Health Disparities
NYU	New York University
OMB	Office of Management and Budget
PCA	principal component analysis
PCORI	Patient-Centered Outcomes Research Institute

PCSK9	proprotein convertase subtilisin/kexin type 9
PEL	Peruvian in Lima, Peru
PERSIAN	Prospective Epidemiological Research Studies in Iran
PGS	polygenic score
PKU	phenylketonuria
PRISMA	Preferred Reporting Items for Systematic Review and Meta-Analysis
PUR	Puerto Rican in Puerto Rico
QBB	Qatar Biobank
RNA	ribonucleic acid
SALL4	spalt like transcription factor 4
TOPMed	Trans-Omics for Precision Medicine
TSI	Tuscans of Italy
UCLA	University of California, Los Angeles
UK	United Kingdom
UKB	United Kingdom Biobank
UMAP	uniform manifold approximation and projection
UN	United Nations
U.S.	United States
WHO	World Health Organization
YRI	Yoruba in Ibadan, Nigeria

Summary[1]

Genetics is the study of heredity, specifically the mechanisms by which traits or characteristics are transmitted from one generation to the next. Because it is applicable to many areas of human life, genetics garners wide interest. Researchers use human genetic information to address a variety of questions about human history and evolution, human biology, diseases, and heritable traits (e.g., height or serum cholesterol). Researchers have frequently used population descriptors as a shorthand for capturing the continuous and complex patterns of human genetic variation resulting from history, migration, and evolution. Of particular concern is the long-standing use of race, and more recently ethnicity, as this shorthand. In humans, race is a socially constructed designation, a misleading and harmful surrogate for population genetic differences, and has a long history of being incorrectly identified as the major genetic reason for phenotypic differences between groups. Rather, human genetic variation is the result of many forces—historical, social, biological—and no single variable fully represents this complexity (see Chapter 1). The structure of genetic variation results from repeated human population mixing and movements across time, yet the misconception that human beings can be naturally divided into biologically distinguishable races has been extremely resilient and has become embedded in scientific research, medical practice and technologies, and formal education. Many elements of racial thinking, including essentialism and biological determinism, have influenced modern thinking around human genetics, to the marginalization of some peoples and the benefit of others.

---

[1] References are not included in this report summary. Citations appear in subsequent report chapters.

Derived from a person's complete set of DNA, genomic information is increasingly easy and inexpensive to produce, and tools to analyze genetic information are widely available. Accordingly, genetic and genomic information has become far more accessible, and research using human genetic data has grown exponentially over the last decade. The use of genetic information is now widespread across biomedical research, and genetics and genomics research is now conducted by a range of investigators across different disciplines, creating a need for clarity and providing an important opportunity to implement substantive changes to the ways population descriptors are used. Clear guidance about the use of population descriptors is needed before mistakes of the past are integrated into this new era of genomics research.

Race and racism have recently gained renewed attention from the U.S. scientific community. Recognition by the U.S. biomedical research community of the need to address the complex issue of population descriptors in genetics research has never been greater. Although the history of prior attempts to address population descriptors in genetics and genomics research—and the lack of notable change—may create some skepticism about the usefulness of another report aiming to create best practices for this complex area, this is a crucial moment to offer concrete guidance to the research community.

STUDY CHARGE

The study sponsor, the National Institutes of Health (NIH), asked the National Academies to conduct a study to review and assess existing methodologies, benefits, and challenges in using race, ethnicity, ancestry, and other population descriptors in genomics research.[2] The statement of task emphasizes the use of appropriate and valid population descriptors in genomics research, and focuses on understanding the current use of population descriptors in genomics research; examining best practices for researchers in the use of race, ethnicity, and ancestry as population descriptors; and identifying how best practices in the use of population descriptors could be widely adopted within the biomedical and scientific communities to strengthen genetics and genomics research.[3] To accomplish this task, the

---

[2] The full statement of task is presented in Chapter 1 along with a discussion of what was in and out of scope.

[3] The statement of task also identified four areas that are beyond the scope of this committee's recommendations: examining the use of race and ethnicity in clinical care; examining racism in science and genomics; examining the use of race and ethnicity in biomedical research generally (e.g., beyond genetics and genomics research); and providing policy recommendations to NIH and government agencies. See the section "What Is the Goal of This Report?" in Chapter 1 for more detail.

National Academies empaneled a committee of 17 members with expertise in population genetics, human and clinical genetics, genetic epidemiology, statistical and computational genetics and genomics, anthropology, sociology, social epidemiology, demography and population statistics, as well as historical, ethical, legal, and social implications research. Given the charge, researchers who use genetic and genomic data are the primary audience for the report, especially the more technical recommendations and best practices (Chapter 5). However, much of the report is intended for a broader audience (see Chapters 3, 4, and 6).

GUIDING PRINCIPLES FOR THE USE OF POPULATION DESCRIPTORS

Human populations can be described according to countless characteristics: urban versus rural, for example, or smokers versus nonsmokers. The use of such descriptors as race, ethnicity, or ancestry, however, focuses on "descent-associated" groups—sets of individuals whose members are thought to share some characteristic that derives from their common origin (see Box S-1 for key terms). Importantly, the inclusion of population descriptors in genomics, and which specific ones to include, must be a deliberate decision because their use has high stakes for ensuring that research benefits society and mitigates against potential harm, such as race-based health inequities.

The committee considered a range of population descriptors, each revolving around a somewhat distinct feature of human difference and thus offering researchers a specific tool that is more appropriate for some uses than for others. Over the course of the committee's work, the following population descriptors emerged as most relevant to the committee's charge: ancestry, geography, ethnicity, indigeneity, and race/racialized groups. To support researchers making reasoned, deliberate choices in their selection of population descriptors, the description and discussion of each demonstrate what these concepts of human difference can—or cannot—capture in genetics studies.

Although some genetics studies have used descriptors like race as proxies for genetic variation, some genetic epidemiologic studies rely on descriptors like race as proxies for cultural beliefs and practices or for shared environments, in the absence of direct measurements of these latter contextual factors. The environment is the complex of physical, social, chemical, and biotic factors that act upon a person or a community and also shape its form and survival. Social context, an attribute of environment, influences behavior and interacts dynamically with biology, including genetics, throughout the life course to affect human health. Given that human genotypes are not randomly distributed across environmental conditions,

BOX S-1
Key Terminology and Definitions

Ancestry: a person's origin or descent, lineage, "roots," or heritage, including kinship.

Environment: the complex of physical, social, cultural, chemical, and biotic factors that act upon a person.

Ethnicity: a sociopolitically constructed system for classifying human beings according to claims of shared heritage often based on perceived cultural similarities (e.g., language, religion, beliefs); the system varies globally.

Genetic ancestry: the paths through an individual's family tree by which they have inherited DNA from specific ancestors. Genetic ancestry can be thought of in terms of lines extending upwards in a family tree from an individual through their genetic ancestors. Shared genetic ancestry arises from having genetic ancestors in common (that is, overlapping lines of ancestry). In practice, shared genetic ancestry is typically inferred by some measure(s) of genetic similarity.

Genetic ancestry group: a set of individuals who share more similar genetic ancestries. In practice a genetic ancestry group is constituted based on some measure(s) of genetic similarity. Once a set is designated as a genetic ancestry group, its members are often assigned a geographic, ethnic, or other nongenetic label that is common among its members.

Genetic similarity: quantitative measure of the genetic resemblance between individuals that reflects the extent of shared genetic ancestry.

Group label: name given to a population that describes or classifies it according to the dimension along which it was identified. An example is *French* as the label for a group identified by its members' possession of French nationality, where *nationality* is the population descriptor.

Population descriptor: a concept or classification scheme that categorizes people into groups (or "populations") according to a perceived characteristic or dimension of interest. A few examples are race, ethnicity, and geographic location, although this is a non-exhaustive list.

Race: a sociopolitically constructed system for classifying and ranking human beings according to subjective beliefs about shared ancestry based on perceived innate biological similarities; the system varies globally.

See Appendix B for further comments, definitions, and citations.

leading to correlations of genetic and environmental effects, and given the extensive evidence for gene-by-environment interactions in experimental organisms, the committee concluded that environmental factors should often be considered alongside population descriptors in genomics research.

Emerging from the mistakes of past and current use of population descriptors is an imperative to transform not only the use of these descriptors but also the field of genomics research. For the recommendations that follow to successfully advance the appropriate use of population descriptors in genetics and genomics research, they must be grounded in ethical and empirical principles that engender trust and drive trustworthiness of research. Accordingly, the committee developed a set of guiding principles that mutually reinforce one another and undergird the recommendations (see Figure S-1). The guiding principles are *respect, beneficence, equity and justice, validity and reproducibility*, and *transparency and replicability* (Chapter 3).

In short, respect for individual and community preferences, norms, and values should inform approaches when determining what population descriptors to use in research. The principle of beneficence calls on researchers to assess how the selection of population descriptors may not only generate potential good but also potential harm and requires consideration of the effect of population descriptors on health equity. A commitment to equity and justice requires determining whether and how the selection and use of population descriptors will produce equitable benefit to avoid reinforcing existing inequities or introducing new ones. Upholding validity and reproducibility requires judicious evaluation of research objectives and assessment of the appropriateness and purpose of including population descriptors. Transparency and replicability include the obligation to provide a clear rationale for the selection and/or use of population descriptors and to explain decision-making processes in an open and accessible manner to both other researchers and research participants, thus enhancing replicability.

Given the dynamic nature of research and the limitations of this report to fully capture the range of possible use cases in future genetics and genomics research, the guiding principles also provide a foundation and common vocabulary for researchers and other relevant parties to engage in future decision making for contexts that may not be addressed directly in this report.

RECOMMENDATIONS FOR THE USE OF POPULATION DESCRIPTORS IN GENETICS AND GENOMICS RESEARCH

Researchers in human genetics and genomics have often struggled with a lack of clear, specific guidance concerning the use of population descriptors. The committee's recommendations are intended to operationalize the

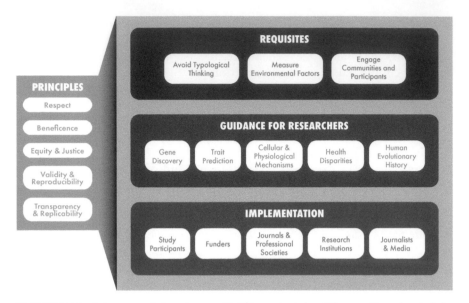

FIGURE S-1 A framework for change. Guiding principles (Chapter 3) undergird the subsequent recommendations, which fall into three categories: requisites for transforming the use of population descriptors in human genomics research (Chapter 4), guidance for researchers conducting different types of genomics studies (Chapter 5), and implementation that includes relevant parties supporting researchers and promoting change throughout the genomics research ecosystem (Chapter 6).

guiding principles with specific practices and procedures to aid researchers. These principles and recommendations offer a starting point for greater harmonization of the uses of population descriptors in genomics research worldwide, without, however, calling for a rigidly standardized approach. The committee does not recommend a standardized nomenclature or typology of population groups, either globally or in the United States alone. The principles and recommendations are intended to provide the basis for a shared approach to grappling with the myriad potential uses of population descriptors in human genomics research worldwide. The recommendations focus on areas that the committee identified as necessary for achieving change, including employing strategies to improve research study design, promoting transparency, tailoring the use of population descriptors for the purpose of a study, and ensuring that researchers have the support needed to implement the recommended best practices.

Requisites for Sustained Change

The committee identified three overarching approaches that are paramount to the long-term success of any effort to resolve the challenging problems surrounding the use of population descriptors in genetics and genomics research: avoiding typological thinking, including environmental factors in study design, and engaging communities. Although not new, these topics warrant increased attention because confronting these challenges could serve as the necessary foundation to catalyze progress.

Avoiding Typological Thinking

Erroneous categorical assumptions can be scientifically and ethically detrimental, particularly when applied to studies of human history, identity, variation, and traits or diseases. There is a pervasive misconception that humans can be grouped into discrete, innate biological categories. The committee cautions against the use of typological categories, such as the racial and ethnic categories established by the U.S. Office of Management and Budget in Statistical Directive 15, for most purposes in human genomics research. While the use of these categories may be required of researchers under certain circumstances (for example, in describing participants in studies receiving federal funding), the fundamentally sociopolitical origins of these categories make them a poor fit for capturing human biological diversity and as analytical tools in human genomics research. Furthermore, use of these categories reinforces misconceptions about differences caused by social inequities. Current practices in human genetics, including the use of descriptors such as continental ancestry, also reinforce these views.

> Recommendation 1. Researchers should not use race as a proxy for human genetic variation. In particular, researchers should not assign genetic ancestry group labels to individuals or sets of individuals based on their race, whether self-identified or not.

> Recommendation 2. When grouping people in studies of human genetic variation, researchers should avoid typological thinking, including the assumption and implication of hierarchy, homogeneity, distinct categories, or stability over time of the groups.

> Recommendation 3. Researchers, as well as those who draw on their findings, should be attentive to the connotations and impacts of the terminology they use to label groups.

- As an example, the term *Caucasian* should not be used because it was originally coined to convey white supremacy,[4] and is often mistakenly interpreted today as a "scientific" term, thus erroneously conferring empirical legitimacy to the notion of a biological white[5] race.
- Another example of a term that should not be used is *black race* because it wrongly implies the existence of a discrete group of human beings, or race, who could be objectively identified as "black."

Although these recommendations help lay the essential groundwork for changing the use of population descriptors, specific guidance for appropriate use is also needed and is provided through subsequent recommendations and best practices.

Including Environmental Factors in Study Design

Genetic effects cannot be adequately explained without nongenetic contexts. In the broadest sense, *nongenetic* or *environment* in gene–environment research refers to everything outside of DNA that influences a person's traits. These factors include physical, chemical, and biological exposures; behavioral patterns, such as sexual practices or physical activity; and social context, such as neighborhoods and income, throughout the life span. Epidemiologic and genetics studies sometimes use race and/or ethnicity as a proxy for cultural beliefs or shared exposures without directly measuring them, even though descent-associated descriptors are not reliable proxies for most environmental factors. Whenever possible, researchers should use variables that more precisely capture the information that is needed to answer the question at hand. Moreover, researchers should not attribute unexplained variance to racial or ethnic differences.

> **Recommendation 4. Researchers conducting human genetics studies should directly evaluate the environmental factors or exposures that are of potential relevance to their studies, rather than rely on population descriptors as proxies. If it is not possible to make these direct measurements and it is necessary to use population descriptors as proxies, researchers should explicitly identify how the descriptors are employed and explain why they are used and are relevant. Genetics and genomics researchers should collaborate with experts in the social**

---

[4] Johann Friedrich Blumenbach (1752–1840) named Europeans *Caucasian* because he felt the most beautiful skull in his collection came from the Caucasus region and was thus a fitting symbol for a superior race (Marks, 1995; Painter, 2010).

[5] The committee chose not to capitalize "black" and "white" throughout the report to recognize and emphasize that they do not signify biological or ethnic groups.

sciences, epidemiology, environmental sciences, or other relevant disciplines to aid in these studies, whenever possible.

As it may not always be possible to directly measure all relevant environmental variables, the committee provides guidance for navigating the associated nuances in later best practices.

Engaging Communities

Communities vary in how individuals and groups self-identify and in their preferences for involvement in a research study. The ways that communities define themselves are dynamic and change over time. Evolving ethical guidelines and frameworks underscore the importance of engaging communities in the research process, in particular by demonstrating trustworthiness and cultivating trust. Effective community engagement improves communication, study coordination, and long-term collaborations between researchers and communities. Conversely, failing to engage and understand communities and relevant parties can undermine trust and trustworthiness of research, diminish public acceptance of the veracity of research results, and importantly, fail to deliver the research outcomes effectively to the communities whom researchers are trying to serve. Effectively engaging communities requires multidisciplinary approaches that draw on expertise in history, sociology, demography, anthropology, communication, and other areas. Research teams should include members with community engagement expertise to better understand how communities identify themselves and discuss the rationale for descriptors or group labels researchers decide to use. Research teams can develop ongoing partnerships with communities by drawing on emerging models and guidelines of community-engaged research.

> Recommendation 5. Researchers, especially those who collect new data or propose new courses of study for a data set, should work in ongoing partnerships with study participants and community experts to integrate the perspectives of the relevant communities and to inform the selection and use of population descriptors.

Guidance for the Selection and Use of Population Descriptors in Genetics and Genomics Research

Because research conducted using genomic data is broad and varied, the committee concluded that there is no one-size-fits-all solution to the challenge of using population descriptors; rather, the appropriate population descriptor depends on the scientific question that is being addressed. Consideration of the different purposes of genetics research gave rise to seven major types of genomics studies, covering both disease and non-disease traits,[6] to serve as a basis for the development of recommended best practices:

1. **Gene discovery for Mendelian traits:** studies aimed at identifying the genetic basis (e.g., pathogenic variant) underlying Mendelian disorders or traits.
2. **Prediction for Mendelian traits:** approaches that rely on the presence of a specific genotype to predict risk for or incidence of a Mendelian disease or specific outcome.
3. **Gene discovery for complex and polygenic traits:** studies aiming to identify genetic variants associated with quantitative traits or complex disease risk, as done in genome-wide association studies (GWAS).
4. **Prediction for complex and polygenic traits:** studies that aim to make probabilistic predictions about individual disease risk or traits based on genomic data.
5. **Elucidation of molecular, cellular, or physiological mechanisms:** studies using related or unrelated participants or cell lines derived from their biological tissues to understand molecular, cellular, or physiological mechanisms.
6. **Studies of health disparities with genomic data:** elucidation of the role of genetic and environmental effects in how social disadvantage leads to health disparities.
7. **Studies of human evolutionary history:** inferences about human evolutionary history using samples of related or unrelated participants.

Responsive approaches are needed both to address the varied types of genomics studies and to accommodate community preferences and evolving conceptions of best practices for grouping individuals and naming those groups.

Transparency in methodology is a scientific norm and the bedrock of replicability, yet the challenge of transparency is one of communicating specifically how and why particular decisions were made—that is, stating the rationale behind the classification scheme and group labels applied when using population descriptors. The lack of both specific practices and transparent reporting can lead to confusion and a lack of comparability among data sets. This lack of transparent reporting could ultimately dimin-

---

[6] Examples are provided in "Classification of Genomics Study Types" in Chapter 1.

ish trust in researchers by those participating in research. Researchers tend to rely on commonly used population descriptors without a clear justification for why they used them. When communicating their research methods, findings, and conclusions, researchers should be as transparent as possible about the specific procedures used to name groups within their data sets. To enhance transparency in reporting, the committee's focus was the conceptual approaches and language that enable appropriate and accurate use of population descriptors in genetics and genomics research. The guidance that follows is intended to provide researchers with feasible best practices and rationales for decision making, in alignment with the guiding principles presented, and is an effort to support the goal of promoting trustworthy research.

> Recommendation 6. Researchers should tailor their use of population descriptors to the type and purpose of the study, in alignment with the guiding principles, and explain how and why they used those descriptors. Where appropriate for the study objectives, researchers should consider using multiple descriptors for each study participant to improve clarity.
>
> Recommendation 7. For each descriptor selected, labels should be applied consistently to all participants. For example, if ethnicity is the descriptor, all participants should be assigned an ethnicity label, rather than labeling some by race, others by geography, and yet others by ethnicity or nationality. If researchers choose to use multiple descriptors, each descriptor should be applied consistently across all individuals in that study.
>
> Recommendation 8. Researchers should disclose the process by which they selected and assigned group labels and the rationale for any grouping of samples. Where new labels are developed for legacy samples, researchers should provide descriptions of new labels relative to old labels.

To better equip researchers with the information to follow these recommendations, the committee developed best practices for different types of genomics studies as well as decision-making tools, including Table S-1 and a decision tree.[7] The research context, including the study type and research questions, gives rise to specific best practices and helps the researcher determine which descriptors apply. Table S-1 suggests which population descriptors are most appropriate as analytical tools for each of the genomics study types outlined in this report. Note that each descriptor represents

---

[7] A full discussion of best practices for each study type is presented in Chapter 5. The decision tree can be found in Appendix D.

a particular *concept of difference* across human populations. The tree and table are not intended to recommend or proscribe specific *words*. Instead, the recommendations in the decision tree and table focus on the conceptual building blocks that researchers should use in study design and data analysis. The objective is to encourage researchers using genomic data to consider, define, and delineate very carefully the concepts of human difference with which they are working.

A nuanced understanding of key terms and concepts is necessary to approach the table and best practices. In this context, *population descriptors* refer to conceptual classification schemes used to group people based on specific characteristics. The appropriate application of descent-associated population descriptors in particular study contexts is the primary focus of the recommendations to follow. Group labels are names given to groupings of individuals. There is the tacit assumption that despite the relative similarity of the individuals within a group the individuals may show variation in other dimensions, including their genetic background.

Many of the best practices recommended by the committee rely on distinctions between genetic ancestry, genetic ancestry *group*, and genetic similarity (Chapter 2). *Ancestry* is a concept encompassing a person's origin or descent, lineage, "roots," or heritage, including kinship. People have an intuitive understanding of ancestry from their family tree, consisting of their biological ancestors (e.g., parents, grandparents, and so forth). The *genetic ancestry* of a person refers to the paths through their family tree by which they have inherited DNA from specific ancestors. *Genetic similarity* between individuals is a quantitative measure of their genetic resemblance, reflective of the extent of their shared genetic ancestry. An analogy may be helpful for elucidating this distinction between a concept (genetic ancestry) and the measures or indicators of that concept (genetic similarity). The concept of wealth is generally understood, but the way it is measured can vary from the amount of money in a person's bank account, to the car they drive, home they own, or sneakers they wear.

Genetic ancestry groups are discrete groups delimited based on one or more measures of genetic similarity. Once demarcated, these groups are typically given a label derived from nongenetic characteristics, including ethnicity, geography, or race. In many contexts, grouping individuals in a study based on genetic similarity alone, without additional labeling, may often be sufficient for the purposes of the study. When choosing to use genetic ancestry or similarity as a population descriptor, careful attention to the intended application is paramount (see best practices in Chapter 5).

As shown in Table S-1, best practices in the use of population descriptors vary by study type. *Careful consideration should be given to whether descent-associated population descriptors are needed at all,* beyond basic descriptions of sampling strategy (e.g., sample collection site and study inclusion criteria). Once researchers identify the appropriate population descriptor for the context of their study, they should then apply group labels consistent with that concept to all study participants. More than one descriptor may be appropriate, and studies may benefit from using multiple descriptors. Finally, population descriptors are sometimes used as proxies for environmental effects (Chapter 2). It should be explicitly noted when population descriptors are used as proxies in this way and the rationale provided. The reader is advised to consult the text in Chapter 5 describing best practices in conjunction with viewing the table. In addition, Table S-1 provides only a broad overview and summary of the best practices; additional considerations for decision making are outlined in a decision tree (see Figure D-1 in Appendix D).

Implementation and Accountability

Despite many previous efforts to provide recommendations, guidelines, and strategies promoting culturally sensitive and valid use of population descriptors, there has been relatively little change in how any entities within the genetics research ecosystem use them. Many aspects of the current systems that fund, support, evaluate, and reward genomics research must change to better facilitate implementation of these recommendations. The genomics research ecosystem has many players, including funders of genetics and genomics research, professional societies, research journals, and research institutions, who all share responsibility for making these changes across an interdisciplinary research community (Chapter 6). Individual researchers bear this responsibility too.

> **Recommendation 9. Funding agencies, research institutions, research journals, and professional societies should offer tools widely to their communities to facilitate the implementation of these recommendations; these tools should be publicly available, especially when they are supported by public funds. Such tools could include:**
> - educational modules for inclusion in human research protection training[8];
> - manuscript submission and review guidelines;
> - grant submission and review criteria;
> - training and education of trainees at all levels;

---

[8] Often called "human subjects" research training. See also https://www.hhs.gov/ohrp/education-and-outreach/human-research-protection-training/index.html

TABLE S-1 Recommended Approaches for the Use of Population Descriptors by Genomics Study Type

This table should be read and interpreted in conjunction with the report text. Consult the decision tree in Appendix D for more information and Chapter 5 text for best practices for each study type. See also the terminology box preceding the table and descriptions of each study type in Chapter 1 section "Classification of Genomics Study Types." For any given study, the use of multiple descriptors may be preferable.

LEGEND

✚	Preferred population descriptor(s)	▬	Should not be used
?	In some cases; refer to Ch. 5 text and the decision tree in Appendix D	E	Descriptors could be used if appropriate proxies for environmental, not genetic, effects

GENOMICS STUDY TYPE	Race	Ethnicity/ Indigeneity	Geography	Genetic Ancestry	Genetic Similarity	Notes
1: Gene Discovery - Mendelian Traits	▬	?	?	?	✚	Similarity suffices as a genetic measure; at fine-scale, other variables may be useful
2: Trait Prediction - Mendelian Traits	▬	E	E	?	✚	No population descriptors may be necessary for analysis
3: Gene Discovery - Complex Traits	▬	E	E	?	✚	Similarity suffices as a genetic measure
4: Trait Prediction - Complex Traits	▬	E	E	?	✚	Similarity suffices as a genetic measure
5: Cellular and Physiological Mechanisms	▬	E	E	▬	?	No population descriptors may be necessary for analysis
6: Health Disparities with Genomic Data	E	E	E	?	✚	Not all health disparities studies rely on descent-associated population groupings, so none may be necessary for analysis
7: Human Evolutionary History	▬	?	✚	✚	✚	Reconstructing genetic ancestry may be of central interest

- opportunities for continuing education for researchers; and
- informatics tools, such as data structure standards for sharing labels and labeling procedures used within a study.

Recommendation 10. Research institutions and funding agencies should embed incentives for fostering interdisciplinary collaboration among researchers with different areas of expertise, including genetics and genomics, social sciences, epidemiology, and community-based research, to facilitate the inclusion of environmental measures and the engagement of diverse communities in genomics research. Funding agencies and research institutions should develop strategies to encourage and reward such collaborations.

Recommendation 11. Given the persistent need to address this dynamic, high-stakes component of genomics research, funders and research institutions should create new initiatives to advance the study and methods development of best practices for population descriptor usage in genetics and genomics research, including the public availability of resources.

Recommendation 12. Key partners, including funding agencies, research institutions, and scientific journals, should ensure that policies and procedures are aligned with these recommendations and invest in developing new strategies to support implementation when needed.

The ability of this report to effect durable change also depends on accountability, which could be enhanced by two mechanisms. First, since both research and social norms will continue to evolve in the future, population descriptors and their use must necessarily change as well. Thus, the committee concluded that it would be valuable to establish multidisciplinary advisory bodies to periodically evaluate current population descriptors and recommend changes based on trusted sociological and scientific data, current cultural norms, and ethical and empirical principles. Second, there is a need for groups with broader powers to monitor and facilitate the implementation of these recommendations.

Recommendation 13. Because the understanding of population descriptors in genomics research is continuously evolving, responsibility for periodic reevaluation of these recommendations should be overseen

by effective, multidisciplinary advisory groups. The advisory groups could:

- periodically reevaluate established best practices on the use of descent-associated population descriptors to ensure they reflect the current state of the science and an ongoing commitment to ethical and empirical principles;
- advise funders and other interested parties on the use of population descriptors and their implementation;
- facilitate the coordination of international best practice sharing;
- provide a venue for input from the broader community, including research participants; and
- monitor and measure changes adopted by funders, researchers, journals, societies, and other relevant parties based on the uptake of best practices identified.

It will take a concerted effort by all relevant parties, patience, and a good bit of time to reach a place where the proper use and reporting of population descriptors is routine and consistent. The recommendations in this report will need to be implemented broadly and consistently, by all the relevant parties, to generate lasting change.

SECTION I

PAST AND CURRENT USE OF POPULATION DESCRIPTORS IN GENETICS AND GENOMICS RESEARCH

SECTION I OVERVIEW

The use of individual and population descriptors in genetics research began with the emergence of human genetics as a science. Despite their importance, historically, such descriptors were never defined, rationalized, used consistently, or standardized. This section explores the early history and context of such descriptors in human genetics, how preferences for certain descriptors have changed over time, and why. Researchers have frequently used descent-associated population descriptors and labels, for individuals or groups, as a shorthand for capturing the continuous and complex patterns of human genetic variation across the globe. Of particular concern is the long-standing and continued use of race, and more recently ethnicity, as this shorthand. Race is a sociopolitically constructed designation, is a misleading and harmful surrogate for genetically based population differences, and has a long history of being incorrectly identified as the major genetic reason for phenotypic differences between groups. Chapters 1 and 2 address this history and consider why these problems have persisted, why another such study is warranted today, and why incorporating different measures of the environment is necessary to improve future genomics studies on traits that involve both genetic and environmental effects.

1

Population Descriptors in Human Genetics Research: Genesis, Evolution, and Challenges

THE STUDY OF HUMAN GENETIC VARIATION

Our social conceptions of race and ethnicity do not match the underlying biological and genetic variation within our species, and we should never confuse the things that were created for the purposes of oppressing people with the nature of that biological and genetic variation.
—Joseph Graves Jr., testimony to the committee
in a public session on April 4, 2022

Genetics is the study of heredity, specifically the mechanisms by which traits or characteristics, known as phenotypes, are transmitted from one generation to the next (King et al., 2014). It is a long-standing observation that no two members of a species, except identical twins or clones, have identical features (Strickberger, 1985), spurring the development of a science that sought to understand how individual traits vary, how this variation is generated, and how it is transmitted to the next generation. This raises the question of how different members of a species can share individual traits, for example, a particular eye color. What is the biological basis of this sharing and its transmission, and is this biological basis the same or different across members of the same species? Since the rediscovery of gene transmission rules in 1900, there has remained a debate on whether such differences and commonalities are from genes, environments, or both, and when there is an effect of genes, whether it stems from one or many genes (Provine, 1971; Provine and Russell, 1986). In recent times, epigenetic and stochastic variation,[1] beyond genetic variation, have been elaborated upon as other causes of phenotypic variation (Panzeri and Pospisilik, 2018).

Human genetics, since its origin in 1900 with the discovery of inter-individual differences in blood transfusions by Karl Landsteiner, has been exceptional among the genetic and genomic sciences in that it focuses on existing groups of individuals to examine heredity rather than only on the offspring of controlled crosses, as is possible in other species. Although the study of trait transmission in human families is widespread and has been successful for rare conditions that follow Mendelian inheritance patterns, family studies are uncommon for common continuous (metrical) pheno-types, whose inheritance patterns are complex or non-Mendelian (NIH, 2007). A more efficient and generalizable study paradigm has, therefore, been to compare and contrast groups of individuals with and without a specific trait feature, such as persons with hypertension versus persons with normal blood pressure. Specifically, what is compared are the frequency differences of a specific genetic variant, this variant being one of at least two forms (alleles) of a gene (Manolio et al., 2009).

Over the past two decades, technological advances have enabled the identification and comparison of genomic sites (base pairs) across the whole genome,[2] both within and outside genes. Regardless of where they are sampled in the world, two human genomes differ at approximately 1 in 1,000 genomic sites on average or a total of 3 million positions (Sachidanandam et al., 2001). While the vast majority of non-ancestral alleles are rare (e.g., found at frequencies of below 1 percent in population samples), most of the variants that differ between two genomes are common and often found in multiple regions of the world (Biddanda et al., 2020; Rosenberg, 2021). The frequency of a variant depends on when it arose, the demographic history of humans who carried it, and whether it affects fitness.

Across the globe, geneticists have catalogued tens of millions of such variants (1000 Genomes Project Consortium, 2015). Most of the common genetic variants existing across human populations arose as early humans evolved within Africa and then migrated across Africa and the rest of the world (Chakravarti, 2014). This variation is a shared human legacy shaping, and in rare circumstances determining, human traits. Studying these variants in, say, hypertensives versus normotensives, can identify variants that are correlated with this trait difference. It takes substantially greater effort to demonstrate whether the detected variants are themselves biologi-

---

[1] Epigenetic variation arises from chemical modification of DNA in body cells (soma), that can modify the functions of genes; not being a permanent DNA change means these are not transmitted to the next generation. Stochastic variation is alteration of gene function from random processes in cells, that are neither genetic nor epigenetic (Angers et al., 2020).

[2] The totality of an individual's DNA is known as their genome.

cal causes of that trait difference or are simply markers that are correlated with the shared history or environment of the individuals studied.

The human population is very young in evolutionary time; when humans are grouped by geographic origin, between-group differences are substantially smaller than within-group differences. Two other historical aspects need to be considered. First, although humans have migrated into new ecologies ever since spreading within and beyond Africa, there has been extensive ancient and recent movement and mixing of peoples both within and across continents, which has affected global patterns of genetic variation (Cavalli-Sforza et al., 1996; Chakravarti, 2014). Second, many humans also have residual ancestry from long-extinct hominids such as the Neanderthals and Denisovans; its extent varies across the globe (Pääbo, 2014).

Human genetic variation is the result of many forces—historical, social, and biological—and cannot be represented by any single variable. Additionally, science is not the only, and sometimes not even the major, source of human origin stories. Each human culture, adapting to its lands and environments over time, has developed its own narrative of its emergence, stories that are rich, powerful, and deeply meaningful to it. The question today is, with all of this knowledge within reach, how should genetics studies of human phenotypes be designed and conducted?

The existence of genetic variation across geographic space does not mean that it is clustered in the distinct groups that notions of race presume. To be sure, if group boundaries on humans are imposed across the globe, thus inventing 2 or 3 or 20 "races," average differences in allele frequencies between geographically distant groupings will be discerned. The existence of such genetic differences in the aggregate, however, is not proof that the boundaries applied were natural, objective, or otherwise genetically meaningful in the first place. Too often, statistical findings of genetic differences between groups are misinterpreted as groupings determined by significant biological/genotypic characteristics as opposed to simply reflecting widespread social presumptions about who is similar to whom based on shared physical/phenotypic characteristics. So, how should individuals and populations be described in genetics and genomics studies? To answer this question, it is crucial to reflect on what such studies aim to accomplish in the first place.

WHAT IS A STUDY USING GENETIC INFORMATION TRYING TO ACCOMPLISH?

Genetic information is assessed directly or indirectly from the genome and can be defined narrowly or broadly. Narrowly defined genetic information is based on data from direct measurements of DNA, RNA, proteins, or epigenetic signatures such as DNA methylation, whereas broadly defined genetic information refers to phenotype information that includes indirect assessments of function (e.g., peripheral blood count) or form (e.g., observable traits such as eye or hair color) influenced by the genome. The advent of the Human Genome Project (HGP) now enables studies of all genes simultaneously using sequence variants across the entire genome. Genetics research typically studies the role of a variant, gene, or small number of genes in an outcome of interest, whereas approaches that interrogate the DNA sequence or epigenetic signatures across the entire genome are known as genomics studies. Both genetics and genomics studies are today common in biomedical research on humans.

Researchers use human genetic information to address a wide variety of questions about history and evolution; the development and function of cells, tissues, and organs; the biology of the human genome; and the risks and mechanisms underlying rare conditions,[3] common and rare diseases,[4] and heritable traits (e.g., height, blood glucose). Genetics and genomics studies are conducted by scientists from a broad range of disciplines (e.g., human and medical geneticists, physicians in various medical specialties, genetic epidemiologists, forensic scientists, evolutionary biologists, biostatisticians, demographers, anthropologists, other social scientists) with different experiences, expertise, and biases. Genetic information is increasingly easy and inexpensive to produce, and tools to analyze genetic information have become widely available and straightforward to use.

Expectations of researchers and the lay public about discoveries made by genetics studies have changed substantially over time. For decades, discovery that a condition or trait had a genetic basis, or more recently, the identification of the specific genetic basis of a condition or trait (e.g., the gene underlying a Mendelian condition such as cystic fibrosis) satisfied both the scientific community and public. However, over the past 10 years, there has been a growing expectation that genetics studies deliver information that can be used for improving health (e.g., accurately estimating the risk of a common disease or accelerating the development of novel treatment approaches and therapeutics) or precisely answering questions about population origins, migration patterns, or the effect of past environmental factors as forces of natural selection. Moreover, information from genetics,

---

[3] In the United States, the Orphan Drug Act defines a rare disease or condition as one that affects less than 200,000 people (21 C.F.R. §316.20(b)); many rare conditions are so-called Mendelian conditions, which means that changes in a single gene are necessary and sufficient to cause the condition (Chial, 2008).

[4] *Common*, beyond frequency, refers to conditions that are variously called polygenic (many genes), multifactorial (many causes), or complex, the latter implying that both genes and environment are causal factors. Examples of such traits are cardiovascular disease, diabetes, and obesity.

genomics, and sociogenomics studies is being used in new ways for financial, political, or legal gain (Bliss, 2020; Roberts, 2011).

Genetics has proven to be a powerful paradigm in medicine, from explaining individual differences in medical outcome (e.g., ABO blood types for blood transfusion and the human leukocyte antigen (HLA) types for organ transplant compatibility), to explaining disease pathogenesis (e.g., in persons with rare Mendelian conditions, such as Marfan syndrome), to identifying therapeutic targets from knowledge of the genes involved (e.g., PCSK9 inhibitors for reducing serum cholesterol). The field has also transformed researchers' knowledge of where and how modern humans arose and migrated across the globe.

Yet, genetics also has substantial limitations. Virtually all conditions and traits are the result of both genetic and environmental factors as well as stochastic or nondeterministic influences. The effect of these nongenetic factors varies across different conditions and traits with some conditions strongly influenced (e.g., susceptibility to infectious disease, obesity, cardiovascular disease) and others only weakly so (e.g., achondroplasia, fragile-X syndrome, Huntington's disease). The effect of nongenetic factors falls between these extremes for most genetic conditions, and the degree to which nongenetic factors influence a condition or trait is itself influenced by the genetic architecture of the condition (e.g., the type, number, and strength of the genetic variants involved), risk genotype(s) (e.g., the variants in an individual's personal genome), and the effect of genetic modifiers (e.g., other genetic variants with indirect influence on the principal genes). Identifying nongenetic factors that influence a genetic condition or trait is challenging, and for most conditions they, therefore, remain unknown. Moreover, without careful study design, the effects of environmental and genetic factors can often be conflated.

It should be further noted that although genetic variation can be critical to identifying disease mechanisms and interindividual trait differences, human biological processes are universal. For example, everywhere in the world, the same ocular biology and neural pathways underlie human vision (Chakraborty et al., 2020). The ingestion of lead produces the same biochemical effects in human bodies whether they are in Alaska or Zambia (Fu and Xi, 2020). Vaccines for coronavirus disease 2019 (COVID-19) work via the same immunological mechanisms in Peru or Poland (Sadarangani et al., 2021). While environmental factors as well as inherited local genetic variants may influence these processes, their physiological mechanisms are essentially the same. In other words, genetic variation is used to identify fundamental mechanisms that are biologically universal among humans— often even relevant to other species, including ones used as model systems (e.g., mice)—to understand human biology and medicine.

CLASSIFICATION OF GENOMICS STUDY TYPES

There is no one kind of genetics or genomics study; thus, it is helpful to consider the various classes of such studies, some of which have a long history of use while others are more recent. Such a categorization is also practical because each study type, with its different questions in mind, recruits study participants differently, and therefore may require tailored guidance to researchers on how to improve the use of population descriptors; in other words, there is no "one-size-fits-all" solution. The committee considers seven such archetypal studies, which are by no means an exhaustive list but serve to illustrate the different usages of population descriptors and highlight some of the considerations that should come into play in choosing a classification scheme for a study:

1. **Gene discovery for Mendelian traits:** studies aimed at identifying the genetic basis (e.g., pathogenic variant) underlying Mendelian disorders or traits.
    -   For a review, see Chong et al. (2015). Examples include the discovery of the cystic fibrosis gene (Kerem et al., 1989), mutations that cause Kabuki syndrome (Ng et al., 2010), or the genetic basis of a trait such as lactose intolerance (Enattah et al., 2002).
2. **Prediction for Mendelian traits:** approaches that rely on the presence of a specific genotype to predict risk for or incidence of a Mendelian disease or specific outcome, as done in research settings or the clinical context of prenatal or newborn screening or presymptomatic testing.
    -   Examples are newborn screening for phenylketonuria (PKU), sickle cell disease, and others (Watson et al., 2022) or analysis of BRCA1/2 mutation-associated tumors (e.g., Shah et al., 2022).
3. **Gene discovery for complex and polygenic traits:** studies aiming to identify genetic variants associated with quantitative traits or complex disease risk, as done in genome-wide association studies (GWAS).
    -   For examples, see case-control studies to identify genetic variants associated with disease risk for type 1 diabetes or Crohn's disease (e.g., Wellcome Trust Case Control Consortium, 2007) or GWAS of height (Lettre et al., 2008).
4. **Prediction for complex and polygenic traits:** studies that aim to make probabilistic predictions about individual disease risk or traits based on genomic data.
    -   Such studies often use "polygenic scores" (also called polygenic risk scores or polygenic indexes; e.g., Khera et al., 2018).

5. **Elucidation of molecular, cellular, or physiological mechanisms:** studies using related or unrelated participants or cell lines derived from their biological tissues to understand molecular, cellular, or physiological mechanisms.
   - Examples include the study of the genetic basis of Huntington's disease (e.g., Kremer et al., 1995) or the cellular mechanism of SARS-CoV-2 infection (e.g., Daniloski et al., 2021).

6. **Studies of health disparities with genomic data:** elucidation of the role of genetic and environmental effects in how social disadvantage leads to health disparities.
   - Examples include kidney disease risk in Hispanics/Latinos and biological aging in children (Kramer et al., 2017; Raffington and Belsky et al., 2022; Raffington et al., 2021; West et al., 2017).
   - It should be noted that not all health disparities studies with genomic data require the use of descent-associated population descriptors. See, for example, a study of genetics and neighborhood effects on health outcomes (Belsky et al., 2019).

7. **Studies of human evolutionary history:** Inferences about human evolutionary history using samples of related or unrelated participants.
   - One example is the study of genomic history of African populations (Fan et al., 2019). For another example, see Waldman et al. (2022).

A series of population descriptors that could be tailored to specific types of genetics studies will be examined in Chapter 2, and best practices for the use of population descriptors will be discussed in Chapter 5 for each of the seven study types.[5]

FEATURES OF HUMAN GENOME VARIATION

By 2001, when the draft sequence of the human genome was reported (Lander et al., 2001; Venter et al., 2001), the tools developed to sequence the human genome and the resulting data were already transforming how genetics research could be done and enabling unprecedented characterization of patterns of human genetic variation (Aach et al., 2001; Birney et al., 2001; Lander et al., 2001). The sequence of the first reference genome was quickly followed by a number of efforts to characterize human genetic diversity such as the International Haplotype Map Project (HapMap),

---

[5] The discussion of other types of genetics and genomics studies, such as those in forensics and genealogy reconstructions, are not a part of this study (see statement of task in Box 1-2).

Genome Aggregation Database (gnomAD), and the 1000 Genomes Project (1000G). These efforts, and the subsequent debates over the sampling and applicability of a limited number of reference populations, led to grappling with the use of population descriptors, specifically race, ethnicity, and ancestry. These projects would confirm the high levels of genetic similarity among humans across the globe and the poor correspondence between racialized groups and the distribution of human genetic variation (Lewontin, 1972). In brief, scientists' current understanding of the distribution of human genetic variation and its evolutionary origins is that

- Anatomically modern humans arose somewhere in the African continent approximately 300,000 years ago (Hublin et al., 2017). Their descendants expanded across much of the rest of the world within the past 100,000 years, giving rise to all modern humans today (Mallick et al., 2016; Nielsen et al., 2017).
- Mating between members of human groups occurred repeatedly throughout evolution, from interbreeding that occurred with archaic forms of humans (e.g., Neanderthal and Denisova) (Narasimhan et al., 2019; Pääbo, 2014), to gene flow between various human groups throughout the world (e.g., Gomez et al., 2014; Reich, 2018).
- Allele frequencies over time and space diverge gradually, owing to random fluctuations (known as genetic drift) and changes caused by natural selection, and are made more similar by gene flow (Novembre and Di Rienzo, 2009). As a result of the relatively recent common origin of modern humans and the repeated mixing of groups, the alleles carried by people living all over the globe show little differentiation:
  - Levels of genetic diversity in humans are low compared to those of many other species: pairs of chromosomes differ only at approximately 1 in 1,000 sites in humans (Leffler et al., 2012), in contrast to 1 in 100 sites in the fruit fly *Drosophila melanogaster* and 3 in 1,000 sites in the chimpanzee (Leffler et al., 2012).
  - Alleles that are common in one population are typically shared across multiple populations, as they tend to be older. Variants that are rare in a population tend to be recent and are usually found much more locally—for example if very rare, only among close relatives (Biddanda et al., 2020).
- Human allele frequencies tend to vary continuously with geographic distance (isolation by distance), with slightly larger differences seen across long-term inhibitors of migration such as oceans

or mountains (Rosenberg, 2021). These geographic boundaries do not correspond to racial groupings.

- Even when differences at any given locus are subtle, information from many loci can be aggregated to make each human genome recognizably unique and to assess an individual's genetic similarity to others (e.g., Figure 2, Novembre and Peter, 2016). This similarity measure is often paired with geographic or other labels from genetically similar individuals in order to assign the individual to a single or multiple groupings (e.g., a method might assign a single geographic population designation or model an individual as a mixture of different "ancestry clusters"; see Chapter 2).

- In some regions of the genome, allele frequencies also vary geographically because a variant contributes to adaption to past or present local environments (Novembre and Di Rienzo, 2009). Where selection on an individual locus was strong and sustained over hundreds of generations, these allele frequency differences can be larger than is typical in the genome. In humans, there are very few cases where one allele is present at very high frequency across a broad-scale geographic region but not shared elsewhere in the world, besides at loci such as those that contribute to infectious disease susceptibility (e.g., the Duffy null allele at the Duffy gene) (Hamblin and Di Rienzo, 2000).

POPULATION CLASSIFICATION SCHEMES IN GENETICS AND GENOMICS RESEARCH

The Origins of Describing Individuals and Populations in Human Genetics

Human genetics research was propelled by the discovery of interindividual differences in blood transfusions by Karl Landsteiner in the early 1900s, and his subsequent demonstration that the bloods of humans can be classified into what we now call the A, B, AB, and O groups (Landsteiner, 1961). Importantly, as early as 1901–1903, he had also suggested that the characteristics that determine blood groups were inherited (Nobel Prize Outreach AB, 2022). Shortly after, in 1910–1911, Emil von Dungern and Ludwik Hirschfeld showed, using families of the teaching staff of Heidelberg University, that Landsteiner's normal human serological features were inherited in a Mendelian pattern (von Dungern and Hirschfeld, 1962), thus making ABO the first known common human genetic trait (Bugert and Klüter, 2012).

In 1919, Ludwik and Hanka Hirschfeld recorded the ABO blood types in more than 8,000 soldiers and refugees on the Macedonian front during

World War I (Hirschfeld and Hirschfeld, 1919). These studies were the first to demonstrate differences in the frequencies of blood group alleles (variants), in mostly unrelated individuals, across different populations whom the authors refer to as "races" (Hirschfeld and Hirschfeld, 1919). The population descriptors used were highly varied and included a mix of continental, geographic, and religious labels (e.g., Europeans, Indians, and Jews). This study on a very large sample of heterogeneous individuals, which also showed geographic patterns of east–west and north–south blood group allele frequency variation, became highly influential in anthropology and human genetics by suggesting widespread allele frequency differences in human populations (Hirschfeld and Hirschfeld, 1919). By 1977, Arthur E. Mourant, a British hematologist and geneticist, had updated his compilation titled *The Distribution of the Human Blood Groups* to include genotype and allele frequency data from hundreds of thousands of samples collected across the globe (Mourant, 1977). These samples were also identified by a dizzying array of terms meant to signify their origin.

The choices of population descriptors used by twentieth-century scientists were consistent with a long-standing European and U.S. belief that human beings are naturally divided into biologically distinguishable races (Gossett, 1997; Hammonds and Herzig, 2009; Keel, 2018; Painter, 2010). The categorization of human beings into races was integral to settler colonialism and slavery, and simultaneously became foundational to scientific thinking in the United States (Frederickson, 2002; Higginbotham et al., forthcoming; Roberts, 2011; Smedley and Smedley, 2012; TallBear, 2013). For example, prominent nineteenth-century scientists such as Harvard biologist Louis Agassiz and Samuel Morton, president of the Academy of Natural Sciences in Philadelphia, promoted the white supremacist view that human beings were divided into unequal racial groups that descended from separate origins (Gould, 1996). These ideas continued to influence U.S. science after the Civil War and persisted through the eugenics era in the twentieth century into the twenty-first century (Graves, 2001; Reardon, 2009; Roberts, 2011; Zuberi, 2003). Some of the harmful scientific and societal practices of the eugenics era are described in a recently released statement and report[6] from the American Society of Human Genetics, acknowledging and apologizing for the involvement of some of its early leaders in the American eugenics movement.

Classifying people by race has been essential to institutional racism and tightly interwoven into political, economic, legal, scientific, and social practices in the United States. Race was "baked into" the very first instruments of governance in the United States, from its first census to its first law governing who could become a citizen (both in 1790). Under the Jim Crow

---

[6] See https://www.ashg.org/wp-content/uploads/2023/01/Facing_Our_History-Building_an_Equitable_Future_Final_Report_January_2023.pdf (accessed January 25, 2023).

regime, which extended from the end of Reconstruction to the Supreme Court's 1954 *Brown v. Board of Education* decision and the passage of federal civil rights legislation, many states maintained rigid racial classification systems to help enforce *de jure* segregation (Dorr, 2008; Pascoe, 2009). The civil rights movement of the 1950s through the 1970s also shaped the scientific use of race, ethnicity, and ancestry as descriptors. New federal legislation, including the Civil Rights Act of 1964, the Voting Rights Act of 1965, the Fair Housing Act of 1968, and the Home Mortgage Disclosure Act of 1975, required many federal agencies to monitor discrimination and to do so meant classifying people, typically into racial and ethnic categories. In 1977, the Office of Management and Budget (OMB) issued Statistical Directive 15–Race and Ethnic Standards for Federal Statistics and Administrative Reporting to standardize federal agencies' recordkeeping, collection, and presentation of data on race and ethnicity (equated with Hispanic origin), including its use on the census (OMB, 1977, 1997).

OMB Directive 15 has had widespread effects because its racial and ethnic categories have been used widely across government and the private sector, including by many scientific researchers in genetics and genomics (Kahn, 2006; Nobles, 2000). This is in part because the NIH and other federal research agencies require OMB-based racial and ethnic information collection in funding proposals and applications for purposes of inclusion (Epstein, 2007). Although OMB Directive 15 is clear that race is a social— and not a biological—classification, this categorization is frequently applied as if it were biological. Thus, the institutional demand for biomedical research to become more inclusive has led to many U.S.-based genetics and genomics research projects collecting OMB ethnic and racial category-based information on study participants, including measurement of biological differences between these groups (Epstein, 2007).

Race and racism also continue to figure in genomics research because many scientists hold the view that race is a biological category or that race is a useful proxy for human biological variation. Scientists not only learn biological concepts of race in their professional training but also, like the rest of U.S. society, are exposed from the earliest ages to racial concepts and practices (Morning, 2011). Racial taxonomy becomes a familiar way of seeing and describing the world, one that is taken for granted and presumed to be "natural" and objective (Hirschfeld, 1996; Hirschfeld and Gelman, 1997; Obasogie, 2010; Van Ausdale and Feagin, 1996). This framework has made its way unnoticed into the design and execution of scientific research. For example, a study by Fujimura and Rajagopalan (2011) highlights how despite the development of new technologies focused on genetic similarity that would preclude the need for pre-labeling populations, the use of terminology such as "ancestry" or "shared ancestry" in genetic analyses can lead to slippage toward racial concepts. In some cases, certain tools and practices currently used in genomics research can blur the differences between ancestry and race (Fullwiley, 2008). In their study of geneticists' population labeling practices, Panofsky and Bliss (2017) found "persistent and indiscriminate blending of classification schemes" that has made the definition of population in genetics "more ambiguous rather than standardized over time" (p. 59). The outsized influence of U.S.-based research on scientific practice worldwide, moreover, means that Americans' widespread exposure to racial thought, discourse, and institutions is transmitted to scientists around the globe.

A complete history of the use of population descriptors in human genetics and the early and persistent use of race in science is beyond the scope of this report and outside of the committee's statement of task. The brief summary provided here is meant only to emphasize several important points. First, early studies, like those by the Hirschfelds, used population descriptors of many categories—racial, continental, ethnic, religious, and more—in ways that imply an interchangeableness among them when none may have existed. Second, the biological concept of race in humans was created to support settler colonialism and slavery, and has always been entangled with racist institutions, policies, and practices. The use of race as a population descriptor in scientific research therefore has caused incalculable confusion and harm. Third, the federal requirement to use OMB categories in many contexts perpetuates the institutional racism, confusion, and harm caused by false concepts of race as a biological grouping. Fourth, racist concepts of race that are deeply embedded in science and U.S. society more broadly continue to affect scientific thinking and research. Scientists must critically examine the underlying assumptions about race—and human commonality and difference—that shape their research studies. For a more complete history of population descriptors in genetics, and for a deeper understanding of the history of the race concept and the intersections of race, science, and society, see the list of references in Box 1-1.

Local and Global Contexts

The conceptualization of "American" as an equivalent to being from the United States has led to the use of derived terms such as *African American*, *European American*, and *Native American*. This terminology has been adopted by the genetics community and applied in many population genomics studies (Bryc et al., 2015; Kidd et al., 2012; Price et al., 2007; Ruiz-Linares et al., 2014; Williamson et al., 2007). However, outside the United States these terms do not have the same context and may imply different meanings, as the adjective *American* has a geographic reach across the North and South American continents, meaning the Americas, rather than a national one (the United States). It is important to move away from

BOX 1-1
Race, Science, and Society: A Reference List

Anderson, Margo J. 1988. *The American Census: A Social History*. New Haven, CT: Yale University Press.

Byron, Gay L. 2002. *Symbolic Blackness and Ethnic Difference in Early Christian Literature*. London: Routledge.

Carter, J. Kameron. 2008. *Race: A Theological Account*. New York: Oxford University Press.

Dorr, Gregory M. 2008. *Segregation's Science: Eugenics and Society in Virginia*. Charlottesville, VA: University of Virginia Press.

Fredrickson, George M. 2002. *Racism: A Short History*. Princeton, NJ: Princeton University Press.

Goodman, Alan H., Yolanda T. Moses, and Joseph L. Jones. 2019. *Race: Are We So Different?* Hoboken, NJ: Wiley-Blackwell.

Gossett, Thomas F. 1997. *Race: The History of an Idea in America*. New York: Oxford University Press.

Gould, Stephen J. 1996. *The Mismeasure of Man*. New York: W. W. Norton & Company.

Graves, Joseph L., Jr. 2001. *The Emperor's Clothes: Biological Theories of Race at the Millennium*. New Brunswick, NJ: Rutgers University Press.

Hammonds, Evelynn M. and Rebecca M. Herzig. 2009. *The Nature of Difference: Sciences of Race in the United States from Jefferson to Genomics*. Cambridge, MA: MIT Press.

Hannaford, Ivan. 1996. *Race: The History of an Idea in the West*. Washington, DC: The Woodrow Wilson Center Press.

Keel, Terence. 2018. *Divine Variations: How Christian Thought Became Racial Science*. Stanford, CA: Stanford University Press.

Marks, Jonathan. 2017. *Is Science Racist?* Cambridge: Polity.

Marx, Anthony W. 1998. *Making Race and Nation: A Comparison of South Africa, the United States, and Brazil*. Cambridge: Cambridge University Press.

Molina, Natalia. 2006. *Fit to Be Citizens: Public Health and Race in Los Angeles, 1879-1939*. Berkeley, CA: University of California Press.

Morning, Ann. 2011. *The Nature of Race: How Scientists Think and Teach About Human Difference*. Berkeley, CA: University of California Press.

Nobles, Melissa. 2000. *Shades of Citizenship: Race and the Census in Modern Politics*. Stanford, CA: Stanford University Press.

Painter, Nell I. 2010. *The History of White People*. New York: W. W. Norton & Company.

Continued

BOX 1-1 Continued

Pascoe, Peggy. 2009. *What Comes Naturally: Miscegenation Law and the Making of Race in America.* New York: Oxford University Press.

Reardon, Jenny. 2005. *Race to the Finish: Identity and Governance in an Age of Genomics.* Princeton, NJ: Princeton University Press.

Roberts, Dorothy. 2011. *Fatal Invention: How Science, Politics, and Big Business Re-create Race in the Twenty-first Century.* New York: The New Press.

Sanders, Edith R. 1969. "The Hamitic Hypothesis; Its Origins and Functions in Time Perspective." *Journal of African History* X:521-532.

Schor, Paul. 2017. *Counting Americans: How the US Census Classified the Nation.* Oxford: Oxford University Press.

Smedley, Audrey, and Brian Smedley. 2012. *Race in North America: Origin and Evolution of a Worldview.* Boulder, CO: Westview Press.

Snowden, Frank M., Jr. 1983. *Before Color Prejudice: The Ancient View of Blacks.* Cambridge, MA: Harvard University Press.

Stepan, Nancy. 1982. *The Idea of Race in Science: Great Britain, 1800-1960.* London: Palgrave MacMillan.

Stern, Alexandra M. 2015. *Eugenic Nation: Faults and Frontiers of Better Breeding in Modern America.* Berkeley, CA: University of California Press.

TallBear, Kim. 2013. *Native American DNA: Tribal Belonging and the False Promise of Genetic Science.* Minneapolis, MN: University of Minnesota Press.

Wilder, Craig Steven. 2013. *Ebony and Ivy: Race, Slavery, and the Troubled History of America's Universities.* New York: Bloomsbury Press.

Yudell, Michael. 2014. *Race Unmasked: Biology and Race in the Twentieth Century.* New York: Columbia University Press.

Zuberi, Tukufu. 2003. *Thicker Than Blood: How Racial Statistics Lie.* Minneapolis, MN: University of Minnesota Press.

U.S.–centric definitions when working with global populations and to be aware of the historical use of alternative descriptors in order to come up with the best possible consensus to embrace diversity while making accurate descriptions of populations for scientific purposes.

Population group classifications are context specific and vary globally. For example, consider the classifications used in ongoing studies from three different countries: the United Kingdom (UK) Biobank, the South African HAALSI study, and the Brazilian BIPMed study (Table 1-1). All population descriptors vary with each study and are not interchangeable. The descriptors are context specific for those regions, and some involve language groups, country of origin, background, or geographic region.

The UK Biobank (UKB) is a biomedical database of genetic and health information from 500,000 participants living in the United Kingdom.[7] The data in the UKB are globally accessible to approved researchers undertaking studies related to health and disease. Thus far, there are over 30,000 global registrations (80 percent from non-UK investigators) (UK Biobank, 2022) and over 5,000 scientific papers published (Conroy et al., 2022). The population descriptors used in the UKB include labels such as *white, mixed*, and so on, as outlined in Table 1-1.

The Health and Aging in Africa: A Longitudinal Study of an INDEPTH Community in South Africa (HAALSI) study includes a community-based cohort of 5,059 men and women 40 years old or older.[8] Study data were collected around the following areas: cognition and dementia, cardiometabolic disease, human immunodeficiency virus (HIV) and treatment, public policies and health, and multimorbidity. While no population descriptor labels are used in the study, data on country of origin were collected (Gómez-Olivé et al., 2018), and in the second wave of the survey, questions related to the languages the participants spoke were included (Berkman, 2020).

The Brazilian Initiative on Precision Medicine (BIPMed) is an initiative of five research, innovation, and dissemination centers funded by the São Paulo Research Foundation (FAPESP) (Rocha et al., 2020). The five centers share data to create BIPMed, which provides genomic and phenotypic information to the global research community. BIPMed investigates the distribution of rare and common variants within two BIPMed data sets including the Brazilian population from the metropolitan area of São Paulo. The Brazilian population structure derives from African, European, and Native American populations (de Moura et al., 2015; Mychaleckyj et al., 2017) but in the BIPMed study, the team decided to use geographic regions where individuals were born as population descriptors as this was more relevant for their study, and it was noted that two regions were not well represented in the data (Rocha et al., 2020).

Challenges with Legacy Data and Harmonization

In an effort to establish uniformity in the use of population descriptors across the globe, several international organizations including the United Nations (UN) and the European Commission have issued recommendations for their member states' census or other data collection efforts related to race and/or ethnicity (Farkas, 2017; UN, 2017). The UN, for example, includes guidance on data collection for ethnic and/or national groups, one of which is to consult with groups that will be categorized. The guidance

---

[7] For more information on the UK Biobank see https://www.ukbiobank.ac.uk (accessed November 3, 2022).

[8] For more information on HAALSI see https://haalsi.org/data (accessed November 3, 2022).

TABLE 1-1 Comparison of Classification Schemes Used in Three Studies Using Genetics from Three Distinct Global Contexts[a]

UK Biobank	HAALSI	BIPMed
White:	Native Language:	Geographic Regions in Brazil
British	Shangaan	where participants were born:
Irish	English	North
Any other white	Afrikaans	Northeast
background	Zulu	Centre West
Mixed	Xhosa	Southeast
White and black	Portuguese	South
Caribbean	Other	Unknown
White and black African		
White and Asian		
Any other mixed		
background		
Asian or Asian British		
Indian		
Pakistani		
Bangladeshi		
Any other Asian		
background		
Black or black British		
Caribbean		
African		
Any other black		
background		
Chinese		
Other ethnic group		
Do not know		
Prefer not to answer		

[a] A more extensive, yet still not exhaustive, list of international programs and the population descriptors they use can be found in Appendix C.
NOTE: BIPMed = Brazilian Initiative on Precision Medicine; HAALSI = Health and Aging in Africa: A Longitudinal Study of an INDEPTH Community in South Africa; UK = United Kingdom.
SOURCES: https://www.ukbiobank.ac.uk; Berkman, 2020; Rocha et al., 2020.

also notes the diversity of categories and terminology across countries and states that "no internationally accepted criteria are possible" as a result (UN, 2017).

Researchers have noted the challenges of harmonization across countries. A study of 138 national censuses conducted around the world in the 1995–2004 period found that 63 percent included some kind of descent-associated question, including those on "race," "population," "tribe," and "caste" (Morning, 2008). In other words, ethnoracial items were far from universal on censuses worldwide. Even among nations that did count their populations by ethnicity or race, they used a wide-ranging set of categories, such as "Kankanaey" in the Philippines or "Rotuman" in Fiji, that did not necessarily overlap with labels used elsewhere. In short, geographic variation in the descent-associated groups that are salient—as well as in the underlying classificatory concepts, practices, and norms that are valued—implies that a single, universal standardization is likely infeasible. In addition, any attempt to impose a standard global framework of population descriptors runs the risk of being detrimental or viewed unfavorably in many locales (Bourdieu and Wacquant, 1999; Onishi and Méheut, 2021; Wimmer, 2015).

Despite the global variation in these systems, in recent years, there has been a growing need in genomics to analyze multiple data sets across studies to increase statistical power and to make cross-study comparisons. However, heterogeneity among studies in their design, recruitment methods, population descriptors, and measurements makes it difficult to easily compare and combine the data and metadata from multiple studies. Challenges of data harmonization include how to deal with missing data or how to compare or aggregate data and metadata in which similar but nonidentical terms are used.

The goal of harmonizing population descriptors is to bring disparate classification systems into greater alignment for specific research goals. Even within a single country, many studies have different recruitment processes and reasons for their selection of population descriptors. Not only are there differences in the specific labels used but also in the underlying concepts represented. In addition, for harmonizing population descriptor data, it is challenging to address across studies differences in scale, resolution, or descriptors used, or to work with studies that use the same term but have different definitions for that term. Existing legacy data often pose additional complications; for example, because some legacy data sets were collected before standards for data sharing were established, there may be uncertainty around whether these data meet current ethical or scientific standards.

As there is no universal system of descriptors, tools and strategies are needed to harmonize them—that is, to reduce heterogeneity—when looking at data across studies. Data harmonization strives to aggregate data from multiple cohorts and/or biobanks to a degree that is scientifically adequate yet acknowledges the heterogeneity among the data sets. There are two main harmonization methods: prospective and retrospective harmonization. Prospective approaches establish standard procedures prior to data collection, making aggregation and comparison considerably easier. One such approach is using common data elements, also called CDEs, which are standardized pieces of information collected as part of a study. However, prospective methods are not always feasible, especially when using existing data sets. Thus, other investigators use retrospective methods to integrate data sets after collection.

ATTEMPTS TO ADDRESS THE USE OF RACE, ETHNICITY, AND ANCESTRY IN THE GENOMIC ERA

Advances in the measurement of human genetic variation and subsequent debates over the sampling and applicability of reference populations have led many in the research ecosystem to grapple with the use of population descriptors, especially race, ethnicity, and ancestry. For more than 20 years, numerous articles have been published and workshops held to discuss these implications, including calls for "a new vocabulary of human genetic variation" (Sankar and Cho, 2002) and the establishment of guidelines for using racial, ethnic, and ancestral categories in human genetics research (Bonham et al., 2018; Caulfield et al., 2009; Flanagin et al., 2021; Khan et al., 2022; NIMHD, 2017; Takezawa et al., 2014; Yudell et al., 2020). Yet, two decades later, use of these descent-associated population descriptors in genetics research remains largely unchanged and controversial.

One impetus for the urgency twenty years ago arose from the rapid technological advancements that made possible whole genome analyses of genetic variation on large numbers of samples. This raised the concern that, without thoughtful guidance, classical and stereotypical views of race and ethnicity would be exacerbated by genome analyses. In 2002, Sankar and Cho published an article on the use of race as a research variable in the study of human genetic variation (Sankar and Cho, 2002). They argued that researchers need to be more thoughtful, deliberate, and precise when designing a study, analyzing the results, and reporting the findings. The authors close their article with an appeal to researchers:

> It is imperative for the research community to acknowledge that the maps used in research are not the only maps used to describe the terrain they study and that careful use of language is necessary to avoid misunderstanding (Sankar and Cho, 2002, p. 1338).

Other studies have focused on why it is difficult to effect change. For example, Caulfield et al. (2009) underscore how researchers work within structures that have been defined by the complex history of race and institutional racism. The obstacles they highlighted were the requirement to use federal directives like the OMB Directive 15 categories of race and ethnicity for reporting; the media's tendency to simplify scientific findings and use race and ethnicity as proxies without explaining how the social categories relate to the research design and results; and the qualities of race, its fluidity, ambiguity, and contingency, which make it difficult to define neatly (Caulfield et al., 2009).

The appropriate use of population descriptors in genomics research is a global issue, not one limited to the United States (Mir et al., 2013). Following a series of workshops held in 2011 and 2012 in Japan, attendees noted that continental labels, such as *European*, *African*, and *Asian*, are tremendously broad, and that among Japanese researchers at the workshop, there was no consensus on what populations should be called Asian. The authors also pointed out, as have others, that when samples are given continental labels but are drawn from limited and specific groups, and there is no attempt to account for the "significant diversity within each region," then the findings may not generalize to the larger group (Takezawa et al., 2014). They closed with recommendations that echo many of those from other researchers around the world, among them

- Respect cultural preferences in labeling processes, and use names that reflect ethnic or cultural backgrounds as much as possible.
- Use categories that are more specific to avoid misinterpretation of results as emphasizing "racial" categories.
- Underscore that genetic and trait differences among populations do not reflect discrete differences but rather frequency or probability.
- Develop a clear summary of research findings to aid journalists in reporting appropriate population descriptors.

In 2016, the National Human Genome Research Institute and National Institute on Minority Health and Health Disparities (NIMHD) hosted a workshop on the use of race and ethnicity data in biomedical and clinical research and how the data are and should be applied to research on minority health and health disparities (Bonham et al., 2018; NIMHD, 2017). A partial summary of the workshop's themes and recommendations includes

- Collect data across multiple dimensions, including self-identified race and ethnicity, race and ethnicity description by others, how individuals perceive others to view their race and ethnicity, self-identified ancestry, and genetic ancestry.
- Update OMB categories, including disaggregating South Asian from other Asian, adding categories to describe individuals from the Middle East/North Africa, adding a category for individuals native to the United States, including an option for multiracial description, adding parent and grandparent self-identified race and ethnicity, including variables to capture sociodemographic data, and updating questions that capture information related to historical racial narratives.
- Educate the public on the purpose of, and misconceptions about, data generated from race-associated biomedical genomics research and distinguish genetic ancestry data from sociopolitical or culturally based racial self-identification. Consider ways to improve clinician and medical student education in human population genetics.
- Work to improve the accessibility and comparability of race and

ethnicity data via the standardization of analysis, tagging, and data reporting; harmonization of methods for data collection, analysis, and reporting; communication of community-based research incorporating race and ethnicity data with study participants; and collaborative efforts to standardize race and ethnicity descriptors in electronic health records (NIMHD, 2017).

In concluding their 2018 paper, Bonham et al. (2018) noted:

> Genomic knowledge has not changed the need to move beyond the misuse of social categories of race and ethnicity as a proxy for genomic variation. The challenge that scientists and medical journal editors must address is how to report human genomic variation without inappropriately describing racial and ethnic groups as discrete population groups (p. 1534).

The National Heart, Lung, and Blood Institute Trans-Omics for Precision Medicine (TOPMed) program collects and analyzes whole-genome sequencing and other -omics data (e.g., RNA, proteins, metabolites) with a wide range of basic and clinical data on heart, lung, blood, and sleep disorders. The program has over 180,000 participants, of whom 60 percent are of non-European descent.[9] TOPMed researchers have recently provided recommendations on using and reporting population descriptors for race, ethnicity, and ancestry in genomics research, including ones that acknowledge the expanding global nature of genomics research and the current focus in the United States on reckoning with racism (Khan et al., 2022):

- Avoid using U.S. racial categories to describe study participants not in the United States.
- Retain detailed population data, if possible, rather than lumping individuals in broader categories early on in the process.
- Understand the potential benefits and harms of analyzing populations before deciding whether to conduct or how to conduct the study.
- Recognize the interdisciplinary work already being done on health care disparities when using these as a justification for genomics research.
- Follow community preference and study-specific reporting guidelines when describing study populations.

---

[9] For more information on TOPMed see https://topmed.nhlbi.nih.gov/ (accessed December 9, 2022).

Despite these and many other efforts, there has been little significant change in the confusing and damaging uses of race, ethnicity, and ancestry as population descriptors in genetics and genomics. In particular, scientists continue to debate whether race is a useful proxy for unmeasured biological differences in human beings—a debate that is fueled by deeply embedded, and often unexamined, biological concepts of race (Nelson et al., 2019; Wagner et al., 2017). Furthermore, scientists are part of a research enterprise whose members (e.g., journal editors, funders, research institutions) to date have failed to effectively coordinate their efforts in developing and implementing transformative policies and practices. Success requires a collective will to confront and resolve the inevitable challenges, change current ways of thinking and doing, and enrich science and society. The committee suggests a path forward in this report.

WHY IS THIS STUDY IMPORTANT?
WHY ANOTHER STUDY? WHY NOW?

While this history of prior attempts to address population descriptors may create some skepticism about the usefulness of another report aiming to create best practices for this complex area, there are several reasons that this is a particularly opportune and important moment to offer concrete guidance to the research community.

Research using human genetic data has grown exponentially over the last decade. Moving from a field largely populated by geneticists, the use of genetic information is now widespread across biomedical research and requires new thinking by all researchers. In addition to a general appreciation of the importance of genetic variation in human disease and health, and the reduction in the cost of and widespread access to genomic technologies, this growth has occurred in part by major investments in large-scale studies, many of which have genomic sequence data available. With this growth, genetics research is now conducted by a wide range of investigators—many of whom have a limited understanding of the rationale and use of population descriptors in human genetics, particularly its history—both exacerbating the risk of misuse of such descriptors and creating an important opportunity to implement substantive changes. Projects such as NIH's *All of Us* Research Program, the Million Veteran Program, and many others will further democratize access to genomic data for clinical research and accelerate this transformation. While some early genetics research included groups of individuals that have relatively high genetic and environmental similarity (e.g., inhabitants of Iceland, Amish residents of the United States) or conducted pedigree studies (Francomano et al., 2003), recent large-scale efforts are enrolling more cosmopolitan and a more diverse set of populations (Morales et al., 2018; Zhou et al., 2022), raising more questions about how best to represent their diversity in the study data. Clear guidance about the use of population descriptors is therefore urgently needed before the mistakes of the past are baked into this new era of genetics research.

With this growth in genetics research has come the development of more advanced methods of understanding and describing population structure and variation, as well as a growing clarity about the contribution of such methods to elucidating the relationship between genetic variation and human traits and health outcomes. Methods to assess genetic similarity and infer genetic ancestry have been developed as have nongenetic approaches, such as geospatial mapping of study participants to states/provinces, cities, and neighborhoods. These advances have been accompanied by the growing recognition of the importance of social and physical environmental factors in health generally, and in modifying the relationship between genotype and disease more specifically (All of Us Research Program Investigators, 2019; Davidson et al., 2022). The importance of these factors has led to new efforts to develop and implement environmental measures in many fields, including in genetics.

These advances have not been accompanied, however, by new approaches to the use of population descriptors in genetics and genomics research. In the absence of a strong and widely disseminated conceptual framework to guide the use of population descriptors, researchers often assume that the only issue is one of finding the "correct" nomenclature for the groups whose data they analyze. This report aims to break new ground by distinguishing on one hand the fundamental conceptual decisions that genetics researchers must grapple with explicitly when they employ population descriptors, from the choices of terminology they face on the other hand. In other words, the committee emphasizes that scientists must get the descent-associated concepts right—that is, have a clear understanding of what these descriptors represent and a rigorous rationale for using them—before selecting the appropriate group categories and labels to work with. Without a deliberate, reasoned, and transparent deployment of population descriptors, human genetics and genomics studies are likely to fall into the same trap as in the past—namely, unwarranted typological thinking that reinforces long-standing prejudices about the characteristics of descent-associated groups.

Since 2020, the U.S. scientific community has become more attentive to the urgency of addressing racism and the lack of diversity in science as well as the admission that little progress has been made in making science accessible and relevant to a more diverse citizenry (Yudell et al., 2020). Research universities embarked on efforts to address diversity, equity, and inclusion in their scientific and educational programs. The social construct of race, the role of intersectionality, and the fundamental effect of racism on all aspects of science and medicine have become parts of faculty trainings at many institutions (Dupree and Boykin, 2021; Holdren et al., 2022; Kossek et al., 2022).

Journal editors recognized the problems of using racial labels in research studies, with growing calls for eliminating the use of high-risk proxy measures (Flanagin et al., 2021; *Nature Human Behaviour*, 2022). The call to remove race from clinical prediction models, like glomerular filtration rate, spread rapidly because of the attention to the danger of false assumptions about innate racial differences and resulting harms to patients (Vyas et al., 2020). Recognition by the U.S. biomedical research community of the need to address the complex and important issue of population descriptors in genetics research has never been greater.

This Report's Audience

Given the charge, the committee notes that the primary audience for the report is researchers who use genomic data. However, the committee recognizes that many of the recommendations and concepts presented in the report will be beneficial to the broader biomedical and social science research communities. One of the foundational tenets of the report is the need for all researchers to be intentional about which population descriptors they choose and how they use and describe descriptors in their research. Furthermore, research is increasingly multidisciplinary; thus, the recommendations in this report could be useful for investigators interested in using biological data that may not necessarily have a genetic component. The chapters of the report reflect the complexity of the task the committee was charged with and the report's diverse audience. Chapter 5 includes a somewhat technical discussion on how to select appropriate population descriptors for genetics research, and there, the primary audience is genetics and genomics researchers. Chapters 3 and 4 focus on guiding principles to support trustworthy research and requisites for change that could facilitate implementation of the recommendations in the report. The committee notes that these two chapters are intended for a more general audience. Finally, to achieve lasting change, the recommended actions in the report will need support from a broad and multidisciplinary group of relevant parties. Chapter 6 includes recommendations for implementation and highlights the roles that study participants; funders of genetics and genomics research; professional societies and research journals; journalists, media, and researchers; and research institutions can play in conjunction with researchers to operationalize the report's recommendations.

WHAT IS THE GOAL OF THIS REPORT?

Given this background, the committee was asked by NIH to review and assess the existing methodologies, benefits, and challenges in using race, ethnicity, and other population descriptors in genomics research (see Box 1-2 for the full statement of task). Fourteen different institutes, program, and offices within the NIH sponsored and funded the study. The statement of task focuses on understanding the current use of population descriptors in genomics research; examining best practices in the use of race, ethnicity, and genetic ancestry as population descriptors; and identifying how best practices in the use of population descriptors could be widely adopted within the biomedical and scientific communities to strengthen genetics and genomics research. The statement of task identifies four areas that are beyond the scope of this consensus study: examining the use of race and ethnicity in clinical care; examining racism in science and genomics; examining the use of race and ethnicity in biomedical research generally (e.g., beyond nongenetic and genomics research); and providing policy recommendations to NIH and government agencies. To accomplish the task, the National Academies convened a committee of 17 members representing diverse expertise areas including human genetics; clinical genetics; population genetics; statistical and computational genetics and genomics; historical, ethical, legal, and social implications research; sociology and anthropology; and demography and population statistics (see Appendix E for the committee biographical sketches).

During the committee's first open meeting, NIH delivered the charge to the committee and clarified information related to the statement of task and the project scope (see Appendix A for the public session agendas). NIH specified that while it would be outside the scope of the committee's work to develop recommendations for the four areas listed in the statement of task as being beyond the scope of this study, discussion and awareness around these topics are necessary to formulate thoughtful recommendations. NIH also clarified that while examining the use of race and ethnicity in clinical care is outside the scope of the committee's work, clinical research using genomic data would be within the scope of the report. Furthermore, representatives said that discussing issues such as the effects of systemic racism in the field of genomics could be a useful context for addressing study design recommendations. NIH also reiterated that the recommendations and best practices identified by the committee over the course of the study would be beneficial for the broader scientific and genomics research communities (as opposed to government agencies) and that the committee should have this audience in mind. NIH acknowledged that the consideration and use of population descriptors is quickly evolving in the scientific community and indicated that it would be useful to identify a framework and principles for considering race, ethnicity, and other population descriptors in genomics research.

The statement of task emphasizes the use of appropriate and valid population descriptors in genomics research. Understanding the potential benefits and harms of past and current population descriptors used in genomics research is discussed at length (see Box 2-1 for key definitions). The committee is mindful that the use of population descriptors including race, ethnicity, and genetic ancestry in genomics research is currently nonstandardized and is influenced by factors such as government categories and journal reporting guidelines. Categories of race and ethnicity, as constructs of social identity and culture, have had long-standing historical implications for individuals in the United States and globally, to the marginalization of some and benefit of others. Genomics research takes place within this context, and social identity from one research participant to the next may vary. The committee is also mindful that additional variation in use of population descriptors is occurring in research studies outside of the United States, and best practices for genomics research might need to be applied differently. See Appendix A for details of the study methods.

BOX 1-2
Statement of Task

An ad hoc committee under the auspices of the National Academies of Sciences, Engineering, and Medicine's Health and Medicine Division will convene to review and assess the existing methodologies, benefits, and challenges in the use of race and ethnicity and other population descriptors in genomics research. The committee work will focus on, but not be limited to, the following tasks:

1. Document and evaluate the variety of population descriptors currently used in genomics research and the potential benefits and challenges of changing these descriptors.
2. Assess how race, ethnicity, and genetic ancestry are currently being used as population descriptors in health disparities research to study genetics and genomics.
3. Assess the appropriate use of race, ethnicity, and genetic ancestry as population descriptors in the determination of genetic risk scores and health risk.
4. Develop feasible and logical approaches to advance appropriate use of race and ethnicity and alternative population descriptors in published genomics research studies.
5. Examine the potential of new, culturally responsive methods and common data elements (CDEs) for advancing harmonization of population descriptors in large genomic studies in the United States and globally.
6. Assess when it is appropriate to use race and ethnicity as population descriptors in genetic and genomic research, and provide recommendations to scientists and researchers for future research.
7. Propose best practices for domestic and international harmonization of population group descriptors.
8. Assess the scientific knowledge of the relationships among race, ethnicity, and population genetic variation.
9. Identify and discuss potential obstacles to implementation of the new methods to describe populations.
10. Discuss potential implementation strategies to help enhance the adoption of best practices by the research community.
11. Identify obstacles and propose best practices in the use of population descriptors with legacy biological samples and associated data.

The final report should describe best practices on the use of race, ethnicity, and genetic ancestry and other population descriptors in genetics and genomics research, as formulated by the committee. Attention should be given to how these best practices could be used by biomedical and scientific communities to increase the robustness of study designs and methods for genetics and genomics research in the United States and globally.

The following elements are beyond the scope of this consensus study:
•   Examining the use of race and ethnicity in clinical care
•   Examining racism in science and genomics
•   Examining the use of race and ethnicity in biomedical research generally (nongenetic and genomics research)
•   Providing policy recommendations to NIH and government agencies

REFERENCES

1000 Genomes Project Consortium. 2015. A global reference for human genetic variation. *Nature* 526:68-74.

Aach, J., M. L. Bulyk, G. M. Church, J. Comander, A. Derti, and J. Shendure. 2001. Computational comparison of two draft sequences of the human genome. *Nature* 409(6822):856-859.

All of Us Research Program Investigators. 2019. The "All of Us" Research Program. *New England Journal of Medicine.* 381(7):668-676.

Anderson, M. J. 1988. *The American census: A social history.* New Haven and London: Yale University Press.

Angers, B., M. Perez, T. Menicucci, and C. Leung. 2020. Sources of epigenetic variation and their applications in natural populations. *Evolutionary Applications* 13(6):1262-1278.

Belsky, D. W., A. Caspi, L. Arseneault, D. L. Corcoran, B. W. Domingue, K. M. Harris, R. M. Houts, J. S. Mill, T. E. Moffitt, J. Prinz, K. Sugden, J. Wertz, B. Williams, and C. L. Odgers. 2019. Genetics and the geography of health, behaviour and attainment. *Nature Human Behaviour* 3(6):576-586.

Berkman, L. 2020. Health and Aging in Africa: A Longitudinal Study of an INDEPTH Community in South Africa [HAALSI]: Agincourt, South Africa, 2015-2019. Inter-university Consortium for Political and Social Research, November 11. https://doi.org/10.3886/ICPSR36633.v3.

Biddanda, A., D. P. Rice, and J. Novembre. 2020. A variant-centric perspective on geographic patterns of human allele frequency variation. *eLife 9.*

Birney, E., A. Bateman, M. E. Clamp, and T. J. Hubbard. 2001. Mining the draft human genome. *Nature* 409(6822):827-828.

Bliss, C. 2020. Conceptualizing race in the genomic age. *The Hastings Center Report* 50 Suppl 1:S15-S22.

Bonham, V. L., E. D. Green, and E. J. Pérez-Stable. 2018. Examining how race, ethnicity, and ancestry data are used in biomedical research. *JAMA* 320(15):1533-1534.

Bourdieu, P., and L. Wacquant. 1999. On the cunning of imperialist reason. *Theory, Culture & Society* 16(1):41-58.

Bryc, K., E. Y. Durand, J. M. Macpherson, D. Reich, and J. L. Mountain. 2015. The genetic ancestry of African Americans, Latinos, and European Americans across the United States. *American Journal of Human Genetics* 96(1):37-53.

Bugert, P., and H. Klüter. 2012. 100 years after von Dungern & Hirschfeld: Kinship investigation from blood groups to SNPs. *Transfusion Medicine and Hemotherapy* 39(3):161-162.

Byron, G. L. 2002. *Symbolic blackness and ethnic difference in early Christian literature.* London: Routledge.

Carter, J. K. 2008. *Race: A theological account.* New York: Oxford University Press.

Caulfield, T., S. M. Fullerton, S. E. Ali-Khan, L. Arbour, E. G. Burchard, R. S. Cooper, B.-J. Hardy, S. Harry, R. Hyde-Lay, J. Kahn, R. Kittles, B. A. Koenig, S. S.-J. Lee, M. Malinowski, V. Ravitsky, P. Sankar, S. W. Sherer, B. Séguin, D. Shickle, G. Suarez-Kurtz, and A. S. Daar. 2009. Race and ancestry in biomedical research: Exploring the challenges. *Genome Medicine* 1(1):8.

Cavalli-Sforza, L. L., P. Menozzi, and A. Piazza. 1996. *The history and geography of human genes.* Princeton, NJ: Princeton University Press.

Chakraborty, R., S. A. Read, and S. J. Vincent. 2020. Understanding myopia: Pathogenesis and mechanisms. In *Updates on myopia: A clinical perspective*, edited by M. Ang and T. Y. Wong. Singapore: Springer, Singapore. Pp. 65-94.

Chakravarti, A. 2014. Perspectives on human variation through the lens of diversity and race. *Cold Spring Harbor Perspectives in Biology* 7(a023358).

Chial, H. 2008. Mendelian genetics: Patterns of inheritance and single-gene disorders. *Nature Education* 1(1):63.

Chong, J. X., K. J. Buckingham, S. N. Jhangiani, C. Boehm, N. Sobreira, J. D. Smith, T. M. Harrell, M. J. McMillin, W. Wiszniewski, T. Gambin, Z. H. Coban Akdemir, K. Doheny, A. F. Scott, D. Avramopoulos, A. Chakravarti, J. Hoover-Fong, D. Mathews, P. D. Witmer, H. Ling, K. Hetrick, L. Watkins, K. E. Patterson, F. Reinier, E. Blue, D. Muzny, M. Kircher, K. Bilguvar, F. Lopez-Giraldez, V. R. Sutton, H. K. Tabor, S. M. Leal, M. Gunel, S. Mane, R. A. Gibbs, E. Boerwinkle, A. Hamosh, J. Shendure, J. R. Lupski, R. P. Lifton, D. Valle, D. A. Nickerson, Centers for Mendelian Genomics, and M. J. Bamshad. 2015. The genetic basis of Mendelian phenotypes: Discoveries, challenges, and opportunities. *American Journal of Human Genetics* 97(2):199-215.

Conroy, M. C., B. Lacey, J. Bešević, W. Omiyale, Q. Feng, M. Effingham, J. Sellers, S. Sheard, M. Pancholi, G. Gregory, J. Busby, R. Collins, and N. E. Allen. 2023. UK Biobank: A globally important resource for cancer research. *British Journal of Cancer* 128:519-527.

Daniloski, Z., T. X. Jordan, H.-H. Wessels, D. A. Hoagland, S. Kasela, M. Legut, S. Maniatis, E. P. Mimitou, L. Lu, E. Geller, O. Danziger, B. R. Rosenberg, H. Phatnani, P. Smibert, T. Lappalainen, B. R. Tenoever, and E. Sanjanade. 2021. Identification of required host factors for SARS-CoV-2 infection in human cells. *Cell* 184(1):92-105.e116.

Davidson, J., R. Vashisht, and A. J. Butte. 2022. From genes to geography, from cells to community, from biomolecules to behaviors: The importance of social determinants of health. *Biomolecules* 12(10).

De Moura, R. R., A. V. C. Coelho, V. d. Q. Balbino, S. Crovella, and L. A. C. Brandão. 2015. Meta-analysis of Brazilian genetic admixture and comparison with other Latin America countries. *American Journal of Human Biology* 27(5):674-680.

Dorr, G. M. 2008. *Segregation's science: Eugenics and society in Virginia.* Charlottesville, VA: University of Virginia Press.

Dupree, C. H., and C. M. Boykin. 2021. Racial inequality in academia: Systemic origins, modern challenges, and policy recommendations. *Policy Insights from the Behavioral and Brain Sciences* 8(1):11-18.

Enattah, N. S., T. Sahi, E. Savilahti, J. D. Terwilliger, L. Peltonen, and I. Järvelä. 2002. Identification of a variant associated with adult-type hypolactasia. *Nature Genetics* 30(2):233-237.

Epstein, S. 2007. *Inclusion: The politics of difference in medical research.* Chicago, IL: University of Chicago Press.

Fan, S., D. E. Kelly, M. H. Beltrame, M. E. B. Hansen, S. Mallick, A. Ranciaro, J. Hirbo, S. Thompson, W. Beggs, T. Nyambo, S. A. Omar, D. W. Meskel, G. Belay, A. Froment, N. Patterson, D. Reich, and S. A. Tishkoff. 2019. African evolutionary history inferred from whole genome sequence data of 44 indigenous African populations. *Genome Biology* 20(1).

Farkas, L. 2017. *Data collection in the field of ethnicity.* Brussels: European Commission.

Flanagin, A., T. Frey, and S. L. Christiansen. 2021. Updated guidance on the reporting of race and ethnicity in medical and science journals. *JAMA* 326(7):621.

Francomano, C. A., V. A. McKusick, and L. G. Biesecker. 2003. Medical genetic studies in the Amish: Historical perspective. *American Journal of Medical Genetics* 121C(1):1-4.

Frederickson, G. M. 2002. *Racism: A short history.* Princeton and Oxford: Princeton University Press.

Fu, Z., and S. Xi. 2020. The effects of heavy metals on human metabolism. *Toxicology Mechanisms and Methods* 30(3):167-176.

Fujimura, J. H., and R. Rajagopalan. 2011. Different differences: The use of 'genetic ancestry' versus race in biomedical human genetic research. *Social Studies of Science* 41(1):5-30.

Fullwiley, D. 2008. The biologistical construction of race: 'admixture' technology and the new genetic medicine. *Social Studies of Science* 38(5):695-735.

Gomez, F., J. Hirbo, and S. A. Tishkoff. 2014. Genetic variation and adaptation in Africa: Implications for human evolution and disease. *Cold Spring Harbor Perspectives in Biology* 6(7):a008524.

Gómez-Olivé, F. X., L. Montana, R. G. Wagner, C. W. Kabudula, J. K. Rohr, K. Kahn, T. Bärnighausen, M. Collinson, D. Canning, T. Gaziano, J. A. Salomon, C. F. Payne, A. Wade, S. M. Tollman, and L. Berkman. 2018. Cohort profile: Health and Ageing in Africa: A Longitudinal Study of an Indepth community in South Africa (HAALSI). *International Journal of Epidemiology* 47(3):689-690j.

Goodman, A. H., Y. T. Moses, and J. L. Jones. 2019. *Race: Are we so different?* UK: Wiley-Blackwell.

Gossett, T. F. 1997. *Race: The history of an idea in America.* New York: Oxford University Press.

Gould, S. J. 1996. *The mismeasure of man.* New York: W.W. Norton.

Graves, J. L., Jr. 2001. *The emperor's new clothes: Biological theories of race at the millennium.* New Brunswick, NJ: Rutgers University Press.

Hamblin, M. T., and A. Di Rienzo. 2000. Detection of the signature of natural selection in humans: Evidence from the Duffy blood group locus. *American Journal of Human Genetics* 66(5):1669-1679.

Hammonds, E. M., and R. M. Herzig (eds). 2009. *The nature of difference: Sciences of race in the United States from Jefferson to genomics.* Cambridge, MA: MIT Press.

Hannaford, I. 1996. *Race: The history of an idea in the West.* Washington, DC: Woodrow Wilson Center Press.

Higginbotham, E., N. R. Powe, G. Barabino, E. Fuentes-Afflick, W. L. Harris, D. S. Massy, E. J. Perez-Stable, R. Pettigrew, P. Pierre, N. Risch, and C. Rotimi. Forthcoming. The use of race in health, science & society: Origins, concepts, implications, alternatives and the path forward. *NAM Perspectives.* Discussion Paper, National Academy of Medicine, Washington, DC.

Hirschfeld, L., and H. Hirschfeld. 1919. Serological differences between the blood of different races: The result of researches on the Macedonian front. *Lancet* 194(5016):675-679.

Hirschfeld, L. A. 1996. *Race in the making: Cognition, culture, and the child's construction of human kinds.* Cambridge, MA: MIT Press.

Hirschfeld, L. A., and S. A. Gelman. 1997. What young children think about the relationship between language variation and social difference. *Cognitive Development* 12(2):213-238.

Holdren, S., Y. Iwai, N. R. Lenze, A. B. Weil, and A. M. Randolph. 2022. A novel narrative medicine approach to DEI training for medical school faculty. *Teaching and Learning in Medicine:*1-10.

Hublin, J.-J., A. Ben-Ncer, S. E. Bailey, S. E. Freidline, S. Neubauer, M. M. Skinner, I. Bergmann, A. Le Cabec, S. Benazzi, K. Harvati, and P. Gunz. 2017. New fossils from Jebel Irhoud, Morocco, and the pan-African origin of *Homo sapiens. Nature* 546(7657):289-292.

Kahn, J. 2006. Genes, race, and population: Avoiding a collision of categories. *American Journal of Public Health* 96(11):1965-1970.

Keel, T. 2018. *Divine variations: How Christian thought became racial science.* 1st ed. Stanford, CA: Stanford University Press.

Kerem, B.-S., M. Rommens, J. A. Buchanan, D. Markiewicz, T. K. Cox, A. Chakravarti, M. Buchwald, and L.-C. Tsui. 1989. Identification of the cystic fibrosis gene: Genetic analysis. *Science* 245(4922):1073-1080.

Khan, A. T., S. M. Gogarten, C. P. McHugh, A. M. Stilp, T. Sofer, M. L. Bowers, Q. Wong, L. A. Cupples, B. Hidalgo, A. D. Johnson, M.-L. M. McDonald, S. T. McGarvey, M. R. G. Taylor, S. M. Fullerton, M. P. Conomos, and S. C. Nelson. 2022. Recommendations on the use and reporting of race, ethnicity, and ancestry in genetic research: Experiences from the NHLBI TOPMed program. *Cell Genomics* 2(8):100155.

Khera, A. V., M. Chaffin, K. G. Aragam, M. E. Haas, C. Roselli, S. H. Choi, P. Natarajan, E. S. Lander, S. A. Lubitz, P. T. Ellinor, and S. Kathiresan. 2018. Genome-wide polygenic scores for common diseases identify individuals with risk equivalent to monogenic mutations. *Nature Genetics* 50(9):1219-1224.

Kidd, J. M., S. Gravel, J. Byrnes, A. Moreno-Estrada, S. Musharoff, K. Bryc, J. D. Degenhardt, A. Brisbin, V. Sheth, R. Chen, S. F. McLaughlin, H. E. Peckham, L. Omberg, C. A. Bormann Chung, S. Stanley, K. Pearlstein, E. Levandowsky, S. Acevedo-Acevedo, A. Auton, A. Keinan, V. Acuña-Alonzo, R. Barquera-Lozano, S. Canizales-Quinteros, C. Eng, E. G. Burchard, A. Russell, A. Reynolds, A. G. Clark, M. G. Reese, S. E. Lincoln, A. J. Butte, F. M. De La Vega, and C. D. Bustamante. 2012. Population genetic inference from personal genome data: Impact of ancestry and admixture on human genomic variation. *American Journal of Human Genetics* 91(4):660-671.

King, R. C., W. D. Stansfield, and P. K. Mulligan. 2014. *A dictionary of genetics.* 8th ed. Oxford University Press.

Kossek, E. E., P. M. Buzzanell, B. J. Wright, C. Batz-Barbarich, A. C. Moors, C. Sullivan, K. Kokini, A. S. Hirsch, K. Maxey, and A. Nikalje. 2022. Implementing diversity training targeting faculty microaggressions and inclusion: Practical insights and initial findings. *The Journal of Applied Behavioral Science* 002188632211323.

Kramer, H. J., A. M. Stilp, C. C. Laurie, A. P. Reiner, J. Lash, M. L. Daviglus, S. E. Rosas, A. C. Ricardo, B. O. Tayo, M. F. Flessner, K. F. Kerr, C. Peralta, R. Durazo-Arvizu, M. Conomos, T. Thornton, J. Rotter, K. D. Taylor, J. Cai, J. Eckfeldt, H. Chen, G. Papanicolau, and N. Franceschini. 2017. African ancestry-specific alleles and kidney disease risk in Hispanics/Latinos. *Journal of the American Society of Nephrology* 28(3):915-922.

Kremer, B., E. Almqvist, J. Theilmann, N. Spence, H. Telenius, Y. P. Goldberg, and M. R. Hayden. 1995. Sex-dependent mechanisms for expansions and contractions of the CAG repeat on affected Huntington disease chromosomes. *American Journal of Human Genetics* 57(2):343-350.

Lander, E. S., L. M. Linton, B. Birren, C. Nusbaum, M. C. Zody, J. Baldwin, K. Devon, K. Dewar, M. Doyle, W. FitzHugh, R. Funke, D. Gage, K. Harris, A. Heaford, J. Howland, L. Kann, J. Lehoczky, R. LeVine, P. McEwan, K. McKernan, J. Meldrim, J. P. Mesirov, C. Miranda, W. Morris, J. Naylor, C. Raymond, M. Rosetti, R. Santos, A. Sheridan, C. Sougnez, Y. Stange-Thomann, N. Stojanovic, A. Subramanian, D. Wyman, J. Rogers, J. Sulston, R. Ainscough, S. Beck, D. Bentley, J. Burton, C. Clee, N. Carter, A. Coulson, R. Deadman, P. Deloukas, A. Dunham, I. Dunham, R. Durbin, L. French, D. Grafham, S. Gregory, T. Hubbard, S. Humphray, A. Hunt, M. Jones, C. Lloyd, A. McMurray, L. Matthews, S. Mercer, S. Milne, J. C. Mullikin, A. Mungall, R. Plumb, M. Ross, R. Shownkeen, S. Sims, R. H. Waterston, R. K. Wilson, L. W. Hillier, J. D. McPherson, M. A. Marra, E. R. Mardis, L. A. Fulton, A. T. Chinwalla, K. H. Pepin, W. R. Gish, S. L. Chissoe, M. C. Wendl, K. D. Delehaunty, T. L. Miner, A. Delehaunty, J. B. Kramer, L. L. Cook, R. S. Fulton, D. L. Johnson, P. J. Minx, S. W. Clifton, T. Hawkins, E. Branscomb, P. Predki, P. Richardson, S. Wenning, T. Slezak, N. Doggett, J. F. Cheng, A. Olsen, S. Lucas, C. Elkin, E. Uberbacher, M. Frazier, R. A. Gibbs, D. M. Muzny, S. E. Scherer, J. B. Bouck, E. J. Sodergren, K. C. Worley, C. M. Rives, J. H. Gorrell, M. L. Metzker, S. L. Naylor, R. S. Kucherlapati, D. L. Nelson, G. M. Weinstock, Y. Sakaki, A. Fujiyama, M. Hattori, T. Yada, A. Toyoda, T. Itoh, C. Kawagoe, H. Watanabe, Y. Totoki, T. Taylor, J. Weissenbach, R. Heilig, W. Saurin, F. Artiguenave, P. Brottier, T. Bruls, E. Pelletier, C. Robert, P. Wincker, D. R. Smith, L. Doucette-Stamm, M. Rubenfield, K. Weinstock, H. M. Lee, J. Dubois, A. Rosenthal, M. Platzer, G. Nyakatura, S. Taudien, A. Rump, H. Yang, J. Yu, J. Wang, G. Huang, J. Gu, L. Hood, L. Rowen, A. Madan, S. Qin, R. W. Davis, N. A. Federspiel, A. P. Abola, M. J. Proctor, R. M. Myers, J. Schmutz, M. Dickson, J. Grimwood, D. R. Cox, M. V. Olson, R. Kaul, C. Raymond, N. Shimizu, K. Kawasaki, S. Minoshima, G. A. Evans, M. Athanasiou, R. Schultz, B. A. Roe, F. Chen, H. Pan, J. Ramser, H. Lehrach, R. Reinhardt, W. R. McCombie, M. de la Bastide, N. Dedhia, H. Blocker, K. Hornischer, G. Nordsiek, R. Agarwala, L. Aravind, J. A. Bailey, A. Bateman, S. Batzoglou, E. Birney, P. Bork, D. G. Brown, C. B. Burge, L. Cerutti, H. C. Chen, D. Church, M. Clamp, R. R. Copley, T. Doerks, S. R. Eddy, E. E. Eichler, T. S. Furey, J. Galagan, J. G. Gilbert, C. Harmon, Y. Hayashizaki, D. Haussler, H. Hermjakob,

K. Hokamp, W. Jang, L. S. Johnson, T. A. Jones, S. Kasif, A. Kaspryzk, S. Kennedy, W. J. Kent, P. Kitts, E. V. Koonin, I. Korf, D. Kulp, D. Lancet, T. M. Lowe, A. McLysaght, T. Mikkelsen, J. V. Moran, N. Mulder, V. J. Pollara, C. P. Ponting, G. Schuler, J. Schultz, G. Slater, A. F. Smit, E. Stupka, J. Szustakowki, D. Thierry-Mieg, J. Thierry-Mieg, L. Wagner, J. Wallis, R. Wheeler, A. Williams, Y. I. Wolf, K. H. Wolfe, S. P. Yang, R. F. Yeh, F. Collins, M. S. Guyer, J. Peterson, A. Felsenfeld, K. A. Wetterstrand, A. Patrinos, M. J. Morgan, P. de Jong, J. J. Catanese, K. Osoegawa, H. Shizuya, S. Choi, Y. J. Chen, and J. Szustakowki. 2001. Initial sequencing and analysis of the human genome. *Nature* 409(6822):860-921.

Landsteiner, K. 1961. On agglutination of normal human blood. *Transfusion* 1(1):5-8.

Leffler, E. M., K. Bullaughey, D. R. Matute, W. K. Meyer, L. Ségurel, A. Venkat, P. Andolfatto, and M. Przeworski. 2012. Revisiting an old riddle: What determines genetic diversity levels within species? *PLoS Biology* 10(9):e1001388.

Lettre, G., A. U. Jackson, C. Gieger, F. R. Schumacher, S. I. Berndt, S. Sanna, S. Eyheramendy, B. F. Voight, J. L. Butler, C. Guiducci, T. Illig, R. Hackett, I. M. Heid, K. B. Jacobs, V. Lyssenko, M. Uda, M. Boehnke, S. J. Chanock, L. C. Groop, F. B. Hu, B. Isomaa, P. Kraft, L. Peltonen, V. Salomaa, D. Schlessinger, D. J. Hunter, R. B. Hayes, G. R. Abecasis, H. E. Wichmann, K. L. Mohlke, and J. N. Hirschhorn. 2008. Identification of ten loci associated with height highlights new biological pathways in human growth. *Nature Genetics* 40(5):584-591.

Lewontin, R. C. 1972. The apportionment of human diversity. In *Evolutionary biology*. Vol. 6, edited by T. Dobzhansky, M. K. Hecht, and W. C. Steere. New York: Springer. Pp. 381-398.

Mallick, S., H. Li, M. Lipson, I. Mathicson, M. Gymrek, F. Racimo, M. Zhao, N. Chennagiri, S. Nordenfelt, A. Tandon, P. Skoglund, I. Lazaridis, S. Sankararaman, Q. Fu, N. Rohland, G. Renaud, Y. Erlich, T. Willems, C. Gallo, J. P. Spence, Y. S. Song, G. Poletti, F. Balloux, G. van Driem, P. de Knijff, I. G. Romero, A. R. Jha, D. M. Behar, C. M. Bravi, C. Capelli, T. Hervig, A. Moreno-Estrada, O. L. Posukh, E. Balanovska, O. Balanovsky, S. Karachanak-Yankova, H. Sahakyan, D. Toncheva, L. Yepiskoposyan, C. Tyler-Smith, Y. Xue, M. S. Abdullah, A. Ruiz-Linares, C. M. Beall, A. Di Rienzo, C. Jeong, E. B. Starikovskaya, E. Metspalu, J. Parik, R. Villems, B. M. Henn, U. Hodoglugil, R. Mahley, A. Sajantila, G. Stamatoyannopoulos, J. T. Wee, R. Khusainova, E. Khusnutdinova, S. Litvinov, G. Ayodo, D. Comas, M. F. Hammer, T. Kivisild, W. Klitz, C. A. Winkler, D. Labuda, M. Bamshad, L. B. Jorde, S. A. Tishkoff, W. S. Watkins, M. Metspalu, S. Dryomov, R. Sukernik, L. Singh, K. Thangaraj, S. Pääbo, J. Kelso, N. Patterson, and D. Reich. 2016. The Simons Genome Diversity Project: 300 genomes from 142 diverse populations. *Nature* 538(7624):201-206.

Manolio, T. A., F. S. Collins, N. J. Cox, D. B. Goldstein, L. A. Hindorff, D. J. Hunter, M. I. McCarthy, E. M. Ramos, L. R. Cardon, A. Chakravarti, J. H. Cho, A. E. Guttmacher, A. Kong, L. Kruglyak, E. Mardis, C. N. Rotimi, M. Slatkin, D. Valle, A. S. Whittemore, M. Boehnke, A. G. Clark, E. E. Eichler, G. Gibson, J. L. Haines, T. F. C. Mackay, S. A. McCarroll, and P. M. Visscher. 2009. Finding the missing heritability of complex diseases. *Nature* 461(7265):747-753.

Marks, J. 2017. *Is science racist?* New York: John Wiley & Sons.

Marx, A. W. 1998. *Making race and nation: A comparison of South Africa, the United States, and Brazil.* Cambridge: Cambridge University Press.

Mir, G., S. Salway, J. Kai, S. Karlsen, R. Bhopal, G. T. H. Ellison, and A. Sheikh. 2013. Principles for research on ethnicity and health: The Leeds consensus statement. *European Journal of Public Health* 23(3):504-510.

Molina, N. 2006. *Fit to be citizens: Public health and race in Los Angeles, 1879-1939.* Berkeley: University of California Press.

Morales, J., D. Welter, E. H. Bowler, M. Cerezo, L. W. Harris, A. C. McMahon, P. Hall, H. A. Junkins, A. Milano, E. Hastings, C. Malangone, A. Buniello, T. Burdett, P. Flicek, H. Parkinson, F. Cunningham, L. A. Hindorff, and J. A. L. MacArthur. 2018. A standardized framework for representation of ancestry data in genomics studies, with application to the NHGRI-EBI GWAS catalog. *Genome Biology* 19(1):21.

Morning, A. 2008. Ethnic classification in global perspective: A cross-national survey of the 2000 census round. *Population Research and Policy Review* 27(2):239-272.

Morning, A. 2011. *The nature of race: How scientists think and teach about human difference.* Oakland, CA: University of California Press.

Mourant, A. E. 1977. *The distribution of the human blood groups.* 2nd ed. Oxford, UK: Blackwell Scientific Publications.

Mychaleckyj, J. C., A. Havt, U. Nayak, R. Pinkerton, E. Farber, P. Concannon, A. A. Lima, and R. L. Guerrant. 2017. Genome-wide analysis in Brazilians reveals highly differentiated Native American genome regions. *Molecular Biology and Evolution* 34(3):559-574.

Narasimhan, V. M., N. Patterson, P. Moorjani, N. Rohland, R. Bernardos, S. Mallick, I. Lazaridis, N. Nakatsuka, I. Olalde, M. Lipson, A. M. Kim, L. M. Olivieri, A. Coppa, M. Vidale, J. Mallory, V. Moiseyev, E. Kitov, J. Monge, N. Adamski, N. Alex, N. Broomandkhoshbacht, F. Candilio, K. Callan, O. Cheronet, B. J. Culleton, M. Ferry, D. Fernandes, S. Freilich, B. Gamarra, D. Gaudio, M. Hajdinjak, É. Harney, T. K. Harper, D. Keating, A. M. Lawson, M. Mah, K. Mandl, M. Michel, M. Novak, J. Oppenheimer, N. Rai, K. Sirak, V. Slon, K. Stewardson, F. Zalzala, Z. Zhang, G. Akhatov, A. N. Bagashev, A. Bagnera, B. Baitanayev, J. Bendezu-Sarmiento, A. A. Bissembaev, G. L. Bonora, T. T. Chargynov, T. Chikisheva, P. K. Dashkovskiy, A. Derevianko, M. Dobeš, K. Douka, N. Dubova, M. N. Duisengali, D. Enshin, A. Epimakhov, A. V. Fribus, D. Fuller, A. Goryachev, A. Gromov, S. P. Grushin, B. Hanks, M. Judd, E. Kazizov, A. Khokhlov, A. P. Krygin, E. Kupriyanova, P. Kuznetsov, D. Luiselli, F. Maksudov, A. M. Mamedov, T. B. Mamirov, C. Meiklejohn, D. C. Merrett, R. Micheli, O. Mochalov, S. Mustafokulov, A. Nayak, D. Pettener, R. Potts, D. Razhev, M. Rykun, S. Sarno, T. M. Savenkova, K. Sikhymbaeva, S. M. Slepchenko, O. A. Soltobaev, N. Stepanova, S. Svyatko, K. Tabaldiev, M. Teschler-Nicola, A. A. Tishkin, V. V. Tkachev, S. Vasilyev, P. Velemínský, D. Voyakin, A. Yermolayeva, M. Zahir, V. S. Zubkov, A. Zubova, V. S. shinde, C. Lalueza-Fox, M. Meyer, D. Anthony, N. Boivin, K. Thangaraj, D. J. Kennett, M. Frachetti, R. Pinhasi, and D. Reich. 2019. The formation of human populations in South and Central Asia. *Science* 365(6457):eaat7487.

Nature Human Behaviour. 2022. Science must respect the dignity and rights of all humans. *Nature Human Behaviour* 6(8):1029-1031.

Ng, S. B.,W. Bigham, K. J. Buckingham, M. C. Hannibal, M. J. McMillin, H. I. Gildersleeve, A. E. Beck, H. K. Tabor, G. M. Cooper, H. C. Mefford, C. Lee, E. H. Turner, J. D. Smith, M. J. Rieder, K. Yoshiura, N. Matsumoto, T. Ohta, N. Niikawa, D. A. Nickerson, M. J. Bamshad, and J. Shendure. 2010. Exome sequencing identifies MLL2 mutations as a cause of Kabuki syndrome. *Nature Genetics* 42(9):790-793.

Nelson, S. C., J. H. Yu, J. K. Wagner, T. M. Harrell, C. D. Royal, and M. J. Bamshad. 2019. A content analysis of the views of genetics professionals on race, ancestry, and genetics. *AJOB Empirical Bioethics* 9(4):222-234.

Nielsen, R., J. M. Akey, M. Jakobsson, J. K. Pritchard, S. Tishkoff, and E. Willerslev. 2017. Tracing the peopling of the world through genomics. *Nature* 541(7637):302-310.

NIH (National Institutes of Health). 2007. *Biological sciences curriculum study.* https://www.ncbi.nlm.nih.gov/books/NBK20363/ (accessed December 8, 2022).

NIMHD (National Institute on Minority Health and Health Disparitie). 2017. *Workshop examines the use of race and ethnicity in genomics and biomedical research.* Bethesda, MD: NIMHD. https://www.nimhd.nih.gov/news-events/features/inside-nimhd/nimhd-nhgri-wrkshp.html (accessed December 2, 2022).

Nobel Prize Outreach AB. 2022. "Karl Landsteiner – facts." *NobelPrize.org.* https://www.nobelprize.org/prizes/medicine/1930/landsteiner/facts/ (accessed November 17, 2022).

Nobles, M. 2000. *Shades of citizenship: Race and the census in modern politics.* Redwood City, CA: Stanford University Press.

Novembre, J., and A. Di Rienzo. 2009. Spatial patterns of variation due to natural selection in humans. *Nature Reviews Genetics* 10(11):745-755.

Novembre, J., and B. M. Peter. 2016. Recent advances in the study of fine-scale population structure in humans. *Current Opinion in Genetics & Development* 41:98-105.

Obasogie, O. K. 2010. Do blind people see race? Social, legal, and theoretical considerations. *Law & Society Review* 44(3-4):585-616.

OMB (U.S. Office of Management and Budget). 1977. *Directive no. 15 race and ethnic standards for federal statistics and administrative reporting.* https://transition.fcc.gov/Bureaus/OSEC/library/legislative_histories/1195.pdf (accessed December 12, 2022).

OMB (U.S. Office of Management and Budget). 1997. *Revisions to the standards for the classification of federal data on race and ethnicity.* https://www.whitehouse.gov/wp-content/uploads/2017/11/Revisions-to-the-Standards-for-the-Classification-of-Federal-Data-on-Race-and-Ethnicity-October30-1997.pdf (accessed December 5, 2022).

Onishi, N., and C. Méheut. 2021. Heating up culture wars, France to scour universities for ideas that "corrupt society." *New York Times*, February 21, 2021.

Pääbo, S. 2014. The human condition—a molecular approach. *Cell* 157(1):216-226.

Painter, N. 2010. *The history of white people.* New York: W.W. Norton & Company.

Panofsky, A., and C. Bliss. 2017. Ambiguity and scientific authority: Population classification in genomic science. *American Sociological Review.* 82(1):59-87.

Panzeri, I., and J. A. Pospisilik. 2018. Epigenetic control of variation and stochasticity in metabolic disease. *Molecular Metabolism* 14:26-38.

Pascoe, P. 2009. *What comes naturally: Miscegenation law and the making of race in America.* Oxford University Press.

Price, A. L., N. Patterson, F. Yu, D. R. Cox, A. Waliszewska, G. J. McDonald, A. Tandon, C. Schirmer, J. Neubauer, G. Bedoya, C. Duque, A. Villegas, M. C. Bortolini, F. M. Salzano, C. Gallo, G. Mazzotti, M. Tello-Ruiz, L. Riba, C. A. Aguilar-Salinas, S. Canizales-Quinteros, M. Menjivar, W. Klitz, B. Henderson, C. A. Haiman, C. Winkler, T. Tusie-Luna, A. Ruiz-Linares, and D. Reich. 2007. A genomewide admixture map for Latino populations. *American Journal of Human Genetics* 80(6):1024-1036.

Provine, W. B. 1971. *The origins of theoretical population genetics.* Chicago, IL: University of Chicago Press.

Provine, W. B., and E. S. Russell. 1986. Geneticists and race. *American Zoologist* 26(3):857-887.

Raffington, L., and D. W. Belsky. 2022. Integrating DNA methylation measures of biological aging into social determinants of health research. *Current Environmental Health Reports* 9(2):196-210.

Raffington, L., D. W. Belsky, M. Kothari, M. Malanchini, E. M. Tucker-Drob, and K. P. Harden. 2021. Socioeconomic disadvantage and the pace of biological aging in children. *Pediatrics* 147(6):e2020024406.

Reardon, J. 2009. *Race to the finish: Identity and governance in an age of genomics.* Princeton, NJ: Princeton University Press.

Reich, D. 2018. *Who we are and how we got here: Ancient DNA and the new science of the human past.* Oxford, United Kingdom. Oxford University Press.

Roberts, D. 2011. *Fatal invention: How science, politics, and big business re-create race in the twenty-first century.* New York: The New Press.

Rocha, C. S., R. Secolin, M. R. Rodrigues, B. S. Carvalho, and I. Lopes-Cendes. 2020. The Brazilian Initiative on Precision Medicine (BIPMed): Fostering genomic data-sharing of underrepresented populations. *npj Genomic Medicine* 5(1):42.

Rosenberg, N. A. 2021. A population-genetic perspective on the similarities and differences among worldwide human populations. *Human Biology* 92(3):135-152.

Ruiz-Linares, A., K. Adhikari, V. Acuña-Alonzo, M. Quinto-Sanchez, C. Jaramillo, W. Arias, M. Fuentes, M. Pizarro, P. Everardo, F. de Avila, J. Gómez-Valdés, P. León-Mimila, T. Hunemeier, V. Ramallo, C. C. Silva de Cerqueira, M. W. Burley, E. Konca, M. Z. de Oliveira, M. R. Veronez, M. Rubio-Codina, O. Attanasio, S. Gibbon, N. Ray, C. Gallo, G. Poletti, J. Rosique, L. Schuler-Faccini, F. M. Salzano, M. C. Bortolini, S. Canizales-Quinteros, F. Rothhammer, G. Bedoya, D. Balding, and R. Gonzalez-José. 2014. Admixture in Latin America: Geographic structure, phenotypic diversity and self-perception of ancestry based on 7,342 individuals. *PLoS Genetics* 10(9):e1004572.

Sachidanandam, R., D. Weissman, S. C. Schmidt, J. M. Kakol, L. D. Stein, G. Marth, S. Sherry, J. C. Mullikin, B. J. Mortimore, D. L. Willey, S. E. Hunt, C. G. Cole, P. C. Coggill, C. M. Rice, Z. Ning, J. Rogers, D. R. Bentley, P.-Y. Kwok, E. R. Mardis, R. T. Yeh, B. Schultz, L. Cook, R. Davenport, M. Dante, L. Fulton, L. Hillier, R. H. Waterston, J. D. McPherson, B. Gilman, S. Schaffner, W. J. Van Etten, D. Reich, J. Higgins, M. J. Daly, B. Blumenstiel, J. Baldwin, N. Stange-Thomann, M. C. Zody, L. Linton, E. S. Lander, and D. Altshuler. 2001. A map of human genome sequence variation containing 1.42 million single nucleotide polymorphisms. *Nature* 409(6822):928-933.

Sadarangani, M., A. Marchant, and T. R. Kollmann. 2021. Immunological mechanisms of vaccine-induced protection against COVID-19 in humans. *Nature Reviews Immunology* 21(8):475-484.

Sanders, E. R. 1969. The Hamitic hypothesis; its origins and functions in time perspective. *Journal of African History* X:521-532.

Sankar, P., and M. K. Cho. 2002. Toward a new vocabulary of human genetic variation. *Science* 298(5597):1337-1338.

Schor, P. 2017. *Counting Americans: How the US census classified the nation.* Oxford: Oxford University Press.

Shah, J. B., D. Pueschl, B. Wubbenhorst, M. Fan, J. Pluta, K. D'Andrea, A. P. Hubert, J. S. Shilan, W. Zhou, A. A. Kraya, A. Llop Guevara, C. Ruan, V. Serra, J. Balmaña, M. Feldman, P. J. Morin, A. Nayak, K. N. Maxwell, S. M. Domchek, and K. L. Nathanson. 2022. Analysis of matched primary and recurrent brca1/2 mutation-associated tumors identifies recurrence-specific drivers. *Nature Communications* 13(1).

Smedley, A., and B. D. Smedley. 2012. *Race in North America: Origin and evolution of a worldview.* 4th ed. Boulder, CO: Westview Press.

Snowden, F. M., Jr. 1983. *Before color prejudice: The ancient view of blacks.* Cambridge, MA: Harvard University Press.

Stepan, N. 1982. *The idea of race in science: Great Britain, 1800-1960.* Palgrave MacMillan.

Stern, A. M. 2015. *Eugenic nation: Faults and frontiers of better breeding in modern America.* Berkeley: University of California Press.

Strickberger, M. W. 1985. *Genetics.* 3rd ed. New York: Macmillan.

Takezawa, Y., K. Kato, H. Oota, T. Caulfield, A. Fujimoto, S. Honda, N. Kamatani, S. Kawamura, K. Kawashima, R. Kimura, H. Matsumae, A. Saito, P. E. Savage, N. Seguchi, K. Shimizu, S. Terao, Y. Yamaguchi-Kabata, A. Yasukouchi, M. Yoneda, and K. Tokunaga. 2014. Human genetic research, race, ethnicity and the labeling of populations: Recommendations based on an interdisciplinary workshop in Japan. *BMC Medical Ethics* 15(1).

TallBear, K. 2013. Native American DNA: Tribal belonging and the false promise of genetic science. Minneapolis: University of Minnesota Press.

U.K. Biobank. 2022. *Apply for access.* https://www.ukbiobank.ac.uk/enable-your-research/apply-for-access (accessed December 5, 2022).

UN (United Nations). 2017. *Ethnocultural characteristics.* https://unstats.un.org/unsd/demographic/sconcerns/popchar/popcharmethods.htm (accessed October 19, 2022).

Van Ausdale, D., and J. R. Feagin. 1996. Using racial and ethnic concepts: The critical case of very young children. *American Sociological Review* 61:779-793.

Venter, J. C., M. D. Adams, E. W. Myers, P. W. Li, R. J. Mural, G. G. Sutton, H. O. Smith, M. Yandell, C. A. Evans, R. A. Holt, J. D. Gocayne, P. Amanatides, R. M. Ballew, D. H. Huson, J. R. Wortman, Q. Zhang, C. D. Kodira, X. H. Zheng, L. Chen, M. Skupski, G. Subramanian, P. D. Thomas, J. Zhang, G. L. Gabor Miklos, C. Nelson, S. Broder, A. G. Clark, J. Nadeau, V. A. McKusick, N. Zinder, A. J. Levine, R. J. Roberts, M. Simon, C. Slayman, M. Hunkapiller, R. Bolanos, A. Delcher, I. Dew, D. Fasulo, M. Flanigan, L. Florea, A. Halpern, S. Hannenhalli, S. Kravitz, S. Levy, C. Mobarry, K. Reinert, K. Remington, J. Abu-Threideh, E. Beasley, K. Biddick, V. Bonazzi, R. Brandon, M. Cargill, I. Chandramouliswaran, R. Charlab, K. Chaturvedi, Z. Deng, V. Di Francesco, P. Dunn, K. Eilbeck, C. Evangelista, A. E. Gabrielian, W. Gan, W. Ge, F. Gong, Z. Gu, P. Guan, T. J. Heiman, M. E. Higgins, R. R. Ji, Z. Ke, K. A. Ketchum, Z. Lai, Y. Lei, Z. Li, J. Li, Y. Liang, X. Lin, F. Lu, G. V. Merkulov, N. Milshina, H. M. Moore, A. K. Naik, V. A. Narayan, B. Neelam, D. Nusskern, D. B. Rusch, S. Salzberg, W. Shao, B. Shue, J. Sun, Z. Wang, A. Wang, X. Wang, J. Wang, M. Wei, R. Wides, C. Xiao, C. Yan, A. Yao, J. Ye, M. Zhan, W. Zhang, H. Zhang, Q. Zhao, L. Zheng, F. Zhong, W. Zhong, S. Zhu, S. Zhao, D. Gilbert, S. Baumhueter, G. Spier, C. Carter, A. Cravchik, T. Woodage, F. Ali, H. An, A. Awe, D. Baldwin, H. Baden, M. Barnstead, I. Barrow, K. Beeson, D. Busam, A. Carver, A. Center, M. L. Cheng, L. Curry, S. Danaher, L. Davenport, R. Desilets, S. Dietz, K. Dodson, L. Doup, S. Ferriera, N. Garg, A. Gluecksmann, B. Hart, J. Haynes, C. Haynes, C. Heiner, S. Hladun, D. Hostin, J. Houck, T. Howland, C. Ibegwam, J. Johnson, F. Kalush, L. Kline, S. Koduru, A. Love, F. Mann, D. May, S. McCawley, T. McIntosh, I. McMullen, M. Moy, L. Moy, B. Murphy, K. Nelson, C. Pfannkoch, E. Pratts, V. Puri, H. Qureshi, M. Reardon, R. Rodriguez, Y. H. Rogers, D. Romblad, B. Ruhfel, R. Scott, C. Sitter, M. Smallwood, E. Stewart, R. Strong, E. Suh, R. Thomas, N. N. Tint, S. Tse, C. Vech, G. Wang, J. Wetter, S. Williams, M. Williams, S. Windsor, E. Winn-Deen, K. Wolfe, J. Zaveri, K. Zaveri, J. F. Abril, R. Guigo, M. J. Campbell, K. V. Sjolander, B. Karlak, A. Kejariwal, H. Mi, B. Lazareva, T. Hatton, A. Narechania, K. Diemer, A. Muruganujan, N. Guo, S. Sato, V. Bafna, S. Istrail, R. Lippert, R. Schwartz, B. Walenz, S. Yooseph, D. Allen, A. Basu, J. Baxendale, L. Blick, M. Caminha, J. Carnes-Stine, P. Caulk, Y. H. Chiang, M. Coyne, C. Dahlke, A. Deslattes Mays, M. Dombroski, M. Donnelly, D. Ely, S. Esparham, C. Fosler, H. Gire, S. Glanowski, K. Glasser, A. Glodek, M. Gorokhov, K. Graham, B. Gropman, M. Harris, J. Heil, S. Henderson, J. Hoover, D. Jennings, C. Jordan, J. Jordan, J. Kasha, L. Kagan, C. Kraft, A. Levitsky, M. Lewis, X. Liu, J. Lopez, D. Ma, W. Majoros, J. McDaniel, S. Murphy, M. Newman, T. Nguyen, N. Nguyen, M. Nodell, S. Pan, J. Peck, M. Peterson, W. Rowe, R. Sanders, J. Scott, M. Simpson, T. Smith, A. Sprague, T. Stockwell, R. Turner, E. Venter, M. Wang, M. Wen, D. Wu, M. Wu, A. Xia, A. Zandieh, and X. Zhu. 2001. The sequence of the human genome. *Science* 291(5507):1304-1351.

von Dungern, E., and L. Hirschfeld. 1962. Concerning heredity of group specific structures of blood. *Transfusion* 2(1):70-74.

Vyas, D. A., L. G. Eisenstein, and D. S. Jones. 2020. Hidden in plain sight—Reconsidering the use of race correction in clinical algorithms. *New England Journal of Medicine* 383(9):874-882.

Wagner, J. K., J. H. Yu, J. O. Ifekwunigwe, T. M. Harrell, M. J. Bamshad, and C. D. Royal. 2017. Anthropologists' views on race, ancestry, and genetics. *American Journal of Physical Anthropology* 162(2):318-327.

Waldman, S., D. Backenroth, É. Harney, S. Flohr, N. C. Neff, G. M. Buckley, H. Fridman, A. Akbari, N. Rohland, S. Mallick, I. Olalde, L. Cooper, A. Lomes, J. Lipson, J. Cano Nistal, J. Yu, N. Barzilai, I. Peter, G. Atzmon, H. Ostrer, T. Lencz, Y. E. Maruvka, M. Lämmerhirt, A. Beider, L. V. Rutgers, V. Renson, K. M. Prufer, S. Schiffels, H. Ringbauer, K. Sczech, S. Carmi, and D. Reich. 2022. Genome-wide data from medieval German Jews show that the Ashkenazi founder event pre-dated the 14th century. *Cell* 185(25):4703-4716.e4716.

Watson, M. S., M. A. Lloyd-Puryear, and R. R. Howell. 2022. The progress and future of US newborn screening. *International Journal of Neonatal Screening* 8(3):41.

Wellcome Trust Case Control Consortium. 2007. Genome-wide association study of 14,000 cases of seven common diseases and 3,000 shared controls. *Nature* 447(7145):661-678.

West, K. M., E. Blacksher, and W. Burke. 2017. Genomics, health disparities, and missed opportunities for the nation's research agenda. *JAMA* 317(18):1831.

Wilder, C. S. 2013. *Ebony and ivy: Race, slavery, and the troubled history of America's universities*. New York: Bloomsbury Press.

Williamson, S. H., M. J. Hubisz, A. G. Clark, B. A. Payseur, C. D. Bustamante, and R. Nielsen. 2007. Localizing recent adaptive evolution in the human genome. *PLoS Genetics* 3(6):e90.

Wimmer, A. 2015. Race-centrism: A critique and a research agenda. *Ethnic and Racial Studies* 38(13):2186-2205.

Yudell, M. 2014. *Race unmasked: Biology and race in the twentieth century*. New York: Columbia University Press.

Yudell, M., D. Roberts, R. DeSalle, S. Tishkoff, and 70 signatories. 2020. NIH must confront the use of race in science. *Science* 369(6509):1313-1314.

Zhou, W., M. Kanai, K.-H. H. Wu, H. Rasheed, K. Tsuo, J. B. Hirbo, Y. Wang, A. Bhattacharya, H. Zhao, S. Namba, I. Surakka, B. N. Wolford, V. Lo Faro, E. A. Lopera-Maya, K. Läll, M.-J. Favé, J. J. Partanen, S. B. Chapman, J. Karjalainen, M. Kurki, M. Maasha, B. M. Brumpton, S. Chavan, T.-T. Chen, M. Daya, Y. Ding, Y.-C. A. Feng, L. A. Guare, C. R. Gignoux, S. E. Graham, W. E. Hornsby, N. Ingold, S. I. Ismail, R. Johnson, T. Laisk, K. Lin, J. Lv, I. Y. Millwood, S. Moreno-Grau, K. Nam, P. Palta, A. Pandit, M. H. Preuss, C. Saad, S. Setia-Verma, U. Thorsteinsdottir, J. Uzunovic, A. Verma, M. Zawistowski, X. Zhong, N. Afifi, K. M. Al-Dabhani, A. Al Thani, Y. Bradford, A. Campbell, K. Crooks, G. H. de Bock, S. M. Damrauer, N. J. Douville, S. Finer, L. G. Fritsche, E. Fthenou, G. Gonzalez-Arroyo, C. J. Griffiths, Y. Guo, K. A. Hunt, A. Ioannidis, N. M. Jansonius, T. Konuma, M. T. M. Lee, A. Lopez-Pineda, Y. Matsuda, R. E. Marioni, B. Moatamed, M. A. Nava-Aguilar, K. Numakura, S. Patil, N. Rafaels, A. Richmond, A. Rojas-Muñoz, J. A. Shortt, P. Straub, R. Tao, B. Vanderwerff, M. Vernekar, Y. Veturi, K. C. Barnes, M. Boezen, Z. Chen, C.-Y. Chen, J. Cho, G. D. Smith, H. K. Finucane, L. Franke, E. R. Gamazon, A. Ganna, T. R. Gaunt, T. Ge, H. Huang, J. Huffman, N. Katsanis, J. T. Koskela, C. Lajonchere, M. H. Law, L. Li, C. M. Lindgren, R. J. F. Loos, S. MacGregor, K. Matsuda, C. M. Olsen, D. J. Porteous, J. A. Shavit, H. Snieder, T. Takano, R. C. Trembath, J. M. Vonk, D. C. Whiteman, S. J. Wicks, C. Wijmenga, J. Wright, J. Zheng, X. Zhou, P. Awadalla, M. Boehnke, C. D. Bustamante, N. J. Cox, S. Fatumo, D. H. Geschwind, C. Hayward, K. Hveem, E. E. Kenny, S. Lee, Y.-F. Lin, H. Mbarek, R. Mägi, H. C. Martin, S. E. Medland, Y. Okada, A. V. Palotie, B. Pasaniuc, D. J. Rader, M. D. Ritchie, S. Sanna, J. W. Smoller, K. Stefansson, D. A. van Heel, R. G. Walters, S. Zöllner, A. R. Martin, C. J. Willer, M. J. Daly, and B. M. Neale. 2022. Global biobank meta-analysis initiative: Powering genetic discovery across human disease. *Cell Genomics* 2(10):100192.

Zuberi, T. 2003. *Thicker than blood: How racial statistics lie*. Minneapolis: University of Minnesota Press.

2

A Multiplicity of Descriptors in Genetics and Genomics Research

INTRODUCTION

Human populations can be described according to countless characteristics: urban versus rural, for example, or smokers versus nonsmokers. With the use of descriptors such as ethnicity, ancestry, or race, however, the focus is on what can be called *descent-based or descent-associated* groupings: populations whose members are thought to share some characteristic that derives from their common origin.[1] Many kinds of classifications fit this bill; *clan, caste,* and *tribe* are other examples. In short, human beings across the globe have devised a family of descent-associated categorization systems (Wimmer, 2013).

As a result, genetics researchers who deem it necessary to incorporate some kind of population descriptor in their work face a choice about which descriptor(s) to use and why. The word *choice* is crucial here because the inclusion of population descriptors in genomics must be a deliberate decision, not a reflex or an afterthought. Groupings of human beings are ultimately cultural constructs that are closely tied to historical and prevailing political, economic, and other conditions, and their use has the potential to have a deep, direct effect on the user's ways of seeing and understanding the social world, specifically as it relates to research participants.

Just as importantly, the many—at times conflicting—social meanings that have been attached to descent-associated groups (for example, prior use of *inferior* or *superior, pure* or *polluted*) have added erroneous con-

---

1 See Hollinger (1998) on "communities of descent," Chandra (2012) on "descent-based attributes," and Morning and Maneri (2022) on "concepts of descent-based difference."

notations to them that impede scientific understandings of human biological variation. Certainly, the parsing of over 8 billion human beings into four color-coded racial categories rooted in ancient Greek humoral theory amounts to an exceedingly blunt tool for describing the human species (Hannaford, 1996). Moreover, the cultural sensitivity of human classification schemes has led to the use of some population descriptors—such as ethnicity and ancestry—as euphemisms for others, notably race, which in turn blurs the conceptual boundaries between them and makes it hard to know exactly what any given descent-associated term is intended to represent.

Accordingly, this chapter presents multiple descent-associated population descriptors and offers a definition of each that delineates it from the others (see Box 2-1 for brief definitions of relevant terms). As members of the broad family of descent-associated concepts, each descriptor has similarities to one or more of the others, yet each also revolves around a somewhat distinct understanding of human difference and thus offers researchers a specific tool that is more tailored for some uses than for others. The committee's objective is, then, to briefly describe the population descriptors that emerged from the study as most relevant to its charge and define them in such a way that scientists and others clearly understand what they can capture—or not—in genetic analyses. Note that these descent-associated measures have a long history of use in genetics, but the rationale for using them has rarely been explicit.

This chapter begins by discussing the concept of ancestry, as it is central to all descent-associated classification and is closely tied to notions of inheritance. Geography is considered next, as it is an equally integral—if less often explicitly recognized—element in the conceptualization of descent-associated groupings. After these two fundamental building blocks, the chapter delves into three population descriptors that are prominent in the United States and which all build on ideas of ancestry and geography: ethnicity, indigeneity, and race. Of note, some of these descriptors have multiple dimensions themselves: geography can refer to place of birth, residence, or ancestral origin; ethnicity might be measured by language, dialect, or religion, for example. Hence it is important to think clearly about the myriad possibilities for population descriptors and make a reasoned, deliberate choice when conducting genomics research.

In addition, this chapter considers the conceptualization and inclusion of environmental variables in human genetics and genomics research. As noted in Chapter 1, most phenotypes are the result of interplay between genetic and environmental factors. Human beings might be categorized, for example, according to their exposure to environmental pollutants and thus their risk for asthma. In other words, environmental factors may lead to the identification of different populations, such as *high risk* and *low risk*, that

BOX 2-1
Key Terminology and Definitions

Ancestral recombination graph: for a set of individuals, the graph depicting the genetic ancestry lines (or paths) that trace back to their common genetic ancestors at every position in the genome.

Ancestry: a person's origin or descent, lineage, "roots," or heritage, including kinship. Examples of ancestry group labels include clan names or patronyms, but geographic, ethnicity, or racial labels are often used to denote groups whose members are presumed to share common ancestry.

Environment: the complex of physical, social, cultural, chemical, and biotic factors that act upon a person.

Ethnicity: a sociopolitically constructed system for classifying human beings according to claims of shared heritage often based on perceived cultural similarities (e.g., language, religion, beliefs); the system varies globally.

Genealogical ancestors: the set of biological ancestors in an individual's family tree or pedigree, including parents, grandparents, great-grandparents, etc. Not all of an individual's genealogical ancestors are their genetic ancestors, that is, have contributed DNA to that focus individual; in fact, most did not.

Genetic ancestry: the paths through an individual's family tree by which they have inherited DNA from specific ancestors. Genetic ancestry can be thought of in terms of lines extending upwards in a family tree from an individual through their genetic ancestors (see Figure 2-1). Shared genetic ancestry arises from having genetic ancestors in common (that is, overlapping lines of ancestry). For a set of individuals, a fundamental representation of genetic ancestry is a structure called an ancestral recombination graph. In practice, shared genetic ancestry is typically inferred by some measure(s) of genetic similarity.

Genetic ancestry group: a set of individuals who share more similar genetic ancestries. In practice a genetic ancestry group is constituted based on some measure(s) of genetic similarity. Once a set is designated as a genetic ancestry group, its members are often assigned a geographic, ethnic, or other nongenetic label that is common among its members.

Genetic similarity: quantitative measure of the genetic resemblance between individuals that reflects the extent of shared genetic ancestry.

Population: a group of humans that is identified by a selected dimension or characteristic (or set of dimensions or characteristics) for the purposes of analysis; this definition does *not* assume that all the group's members are identical or homogenous.

Population descriptor: a concept or classification scheme that categorizes people into groups (or "populations") according to a perceived characteristic or dimension of interest. A few examples are race, ethnicity, and geographic location, although this is a non-exhaustive list.

Continued

BOX 2-1 Continued

Race: a sociopolitically constructed system for classifying and ranking human beings according to subjective beliefs about shared ancestry based on perceived innate biological similarities; the system varies globally.

See Appendix B for further comments, definitions, and citations.

---

researchers consider meaningful for their analyses. Although environmental factors are distinct from genetic ones, their joint and interactive effects on phenotypes compel us to consider them simultaneously. The final section of this chapter explores the inclusion of environmental variables in genetics research, which could be used independently or along with other descriptors.

A RANGE OF DESCENT-ASSOCIATED
POPULATION DESCRIPTORS

Ancestry

Each person has a family tree, a set of biological ancestors consisting of their parents, grandparents, great-grandparents, and so forth. These recent *genealogical ancestors* are often of interest for their sociocultural and biological heritage. Going back in time, their number rapidly balloons and, because there have been only so many people on the planet, the genealogical ancestors of one person quickly begin to overlap with those of another (Figure 2-1). By several thousands of years ago, all modern humans likely share all their genealogical ancestors (Rohde et al., 2004). In other words, modern humans are all embedded within the same enormous family tree, with some members more closely related than others (Figure 2-1).

For a given individual, most of their remote genealogical ancestors did not transmit DNA to them. In fact, only a tiny subset of a person's genealogical ancestors many generations back are also their *genetic ancestors* contributing DNA. At a given position in the genome, a person carries two copies of DNA, inherited from only two of their many genealogical ancestors: for example, they might carry their paternal grandfather and their maternal grandmother's DNA. Which genealogical ancestors contributed DNA changes along the genome. These changes result from two processes: the fact that only half of the genetic material of a parent is transmitted to an offspring and because the transmitted material is itself the result of recombining the parental DNA. Each person's genome is thus a mosaic of DNA segments inherited from a small subset of genealogical ancestors (Donnelly, 1983).

As a result, a person's genetic ancestry can be thought of in terms of lines extending upwards from one ancestor to another in the family tree (see Figure 2-1). From one position in the genome to another, these lines through the family tree will differ, owing to recombination, traversing a distinct succession of genealogical ancestors. When comparing the genetic ancestry of two individuals, the lines of inheritance will coalesce quickly at some positions and remain distinct for longer times at others (Hudson, 1990; Wohns et al., 2022). Segments of the genome inherited by two or more people from the same relatively recent ancestor are referred to as "identical-by-descent" (Thompson, 2013).

Individuals in greater geographic proximity will tend to share more lines of ancestry through their family tree (Coop Lab, 2017b). Eventually, all modern humans will share a genetic common ancestor at any given position in the genome. For a set of individuals, the genetic ancestry lines that trace to the common ancestor at every position in the genome comprise the *ancestral recombination graph* (Hudson, 1990; Schaefer et al., 2021), which can also be understood as a sequence of inheritance paths, called gene "trees" for each segment of the genome (Kelleher et al., 2016; Wiuf and Hein, 1999) (see Figure 2-1 inset). The genetic ancestries of all humans today, no matter how or where they are identified, are embedded within this giant graph.

As this brief summary clarifies, any description of the genetic ancestry of an individual entails a decision about the relevant time depth at which to describe it. For example, given the repeated mixing and long-range migrations that have characterized all human evolution (Reich, 2018), individuals living in close proximity in Europe today, who might be characterized as of some particular regional ancestry or of "European ancestry," trace much of their genetic ancestry also to both central Asia and the Middle East only 8,000 years ago (Haak et al., 2015), and farther back in the past their genetic ancestors lived in Africa (Wohns et al., 2022). Therefore, referring to people with recent genealogical or genetic ancestors in Europe as "white" or of "European ancestry" and people with recent genealogical ancestors in Africa and often Europe as "black" or of "African ancestry" is incomplete, incorrect, and misleading. Similarly, any geographic or ethnic labeling requires that decisions be made about the appropriate level of resolution necessary for a study. In many current studies, individuals have been defined in terms of continental ancestry on a timeframe before the past 600 years, e.g., before the onset of European global colonialism and its associated voluntary and forced population movements, admixture, and the large-scale institution of enslavement.

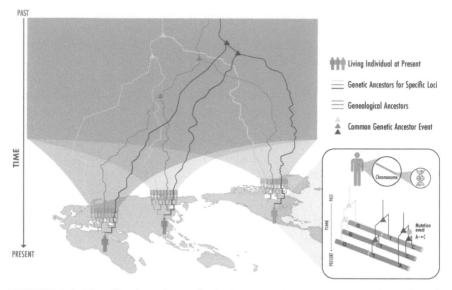

FIGURE 2-1 Visualization of genealogical vs. genetic ancestry. *Genealogical* (pedigree) *ancestors* over time are shown as family tree structures extending into the past (upward) for three present-day individuals sampled from different places around the world. Only a subset of genealogical ancestors contributes genetic material to the living individuals; these *genetic ancestors* and the lines of genetic transmission connecting them are indicated with bolded lines (yellow, green, red) for three exemplar genetic loci (see also inset). Moving back in time, all three individuals eventually share their genealogical ancestors and their genetic ancestors. As indicated, the overlap between family trees that indicate genealogical ancestors happens much more recently than the common ancestor events in the "gene trees" that describe the relationship of genetic ancestors. Who is most closely related genetically to whom varies along a genome, as shown in the inset panel. The inset also demonstrates how mutations that occurred in the past, during the transmission of DNA from one generation to the next, lead to observable changes in DNA today and result in greater or less observed genetic similarity between individuals.

These difficulties are compounded when ascribing population descriptors to groups, as boundaries need to be imposed to divide into bins people who share both genealogical and genetic ancestors. A common approach is to define genetic ancestry groups by first forming clusters of individuals of sufficient genetic similarity based on some genetic measure (e.g., using ancestry proportion inference, see Rosenberg et al., 2002, or principal component analysis, see Reich et al., 2008). These genetic groupings are often then labeled by reference to a nongenetic property that is common in the group, such as a particular geographical origin or ethnicity. Much of the challenge of population descriptors arises from this practice of associating nongenetic terms to clusters of genetically similar individuals and doing so inconsistently within and between studies.

The population descriptors by which individuals are grouped some-times derive from conceptual constructs used in statistical models. For instance, many statistical methods to infer clusters or groups posit the existence of discrete populations with distinct patterns of genetic varia-tion from which individuals derive their genetic ancestry (Pritchard et al., 2000). For analytic convenience, these populations are often assumed to be unstructured, randomly mating groups of individuals, even when such conditions are rarely met in reality. When assuming discrete populations, it may be difficult to model an individual's ancestry as arising from a single population; individuals that are modeled as having ancestry from more than one population are often labeled as "admixed" (Falush et al., 2003; Pritchard et al., 2000). Similarly, when a set of individuals is inferred as deriving ancestry from more than one population, that group is sometimes described as an "admixed population," although individuals within that group may and often do have different degrees of admixture (Lipson et al., 2013; Patterson et al., 2012; Pickrell and Pritchard, 2012).

The concept of admixture carries with it a number of conceptual and interpretive challenges. On one hand, it may be useful for reflecting when an individual or population has lines of ancestry that trace back to multiple distant geographic origins on a recent timescale: for example, in describ-ing individuals from Central and South America whose ancestry 600 years ago traces to individuals mostly living in western Europe, west Africa, and Central/South America. A difficulty, however, is the often-implicit assump-tion of timescale. All humans are admixed, in the sense of having genetic ancestors that lived in different geographic regions at different times. But not everyone is recently admixed: for some, ancestry lines will trace back to geographically distant ancestors within a few generations whereas for others, the same process occurs on a longer timescale. A further challenge is that admixture is almost always framed in terms of modeling constructs of "source populations," which may erroneously imply the existence of homogeneous populations in the past. An example of the problem is when describing individuals as admixed between African and European ances-tries, when neither label refers to a genetically homogeneous grouping or one that is well defined or even stable over evolutionary time. Thus, an unexamined discussion of admixture can lend itself to racialized thinking. The persistence of such thinking in genetics owes in part to the fact that ad-mixture models have been useful in genetic disease mapping (Chakraborty and Weiss, 1986; Freedman et al., 2006; Pritchard et al., 2000): the models are approximately correct for gene mapping despite the assumptions being precisely wrong.

While genetic ancestry is often the descriptive framing used by research-ers to describe individuals or groups in their samples, "most statements about ancestry are really statements about genetic similarity" (Coop, 2022; Mathieson and Scally, 2020). Individuals that share more paths through the family tree will have accumulated fewer genetic differences between them, and thus on average will have more similar genotypes. This genetic similarity is observable using genotyping and sequencing technologies, and so direct observations of genetic similarity provide an indirect reflection of the ancestral recombination graph and the family trees in which it is embedded (see Figure 2-1 inset). Genetic similarity is thus informative about genetic ancestry and, to a much lesser extent, genealogical ancestry, but the relationship among the three concepts is complicated (Coop, 2022; Coop Lab, 2017a) (see Figure 2-1). Moreover, in practice, researchers are often interested only in genetic similarity—such as when assembling study participants for a genome-wide association study—rather than in ancestry over different time periods, and use ancestry labels only as shorthand, at the risk of considerable confusion.

Geography

In surveys of human genetic diversity, a broad correlation is typically observed between genome-wide genetic similarity and geographic proximity (Rosenberg, 2021). It is no surprise then that ancestry, whether genetic or genealogical, is often expressed in terms of geography. The "origins" or "roots" ascribed to people are routinely denoted by geographic labels, using for example, continents or continental regions, such as *European* or *North African*, or political territorial labels at the resolution of a participant's country of origin, such as *Brazilian* or *Japanese*. Geographic proximity is also a crude surrogate for shared environment in studies of ongoing and/ or past exposures to environmental factors, whether biotic (such as pathogens) or abiotic (such as solar incidence). Geographic labels thus frequently attribute shared environmental experiences to groups, even when it is the individual exposures that are relevant to understanding traits. In sum, geography is a widely used population descriptor that stands in for more than one concept of human difference. Indeed, part of its methodological appeal may lie in its seeming to obviate making difficult choices, such as if and how to ascribe ethnic labels to individuals.

Yet geography as a population descriptor presents challenges, many of which are similar to those related to genetic ancestry, such as questions of spatial and temporal resolution. For one, geography is a broad concept that can variously be measured by breaking it down into more precise indicators, such as an individual's birthplace, their current place of residence, or the full trajectory of the locations they have lived. Alternatively, and especially in genetics, the interest may be in the descent-associated notion of *geographical ancestry*, that is, where an individual's genealogical ancestors lived at some time point in the past. Geographical ancestry, like genetic ancestry, thus requires having to specify a timescale. A common approach is to use data from parental or grandparental birthplaces to indicate geographical ancestry one or two generations into the past (Fujimura and Rajagopalan, 2011).

Regardless of the precise geographic location of interest, one common challenge when using geographic population descriptors is how to describe locations. While latitude and longitude can be used in plots and maps, often in a genetics or genomics study, a researcher may wish to find place names to describe a set of geographical locations concisely. This raises the question of how to bin geographic locations together into labels. Various approaches are taken, from using contemporary or past borders of political entities, to referring to features of physical geography. This decision process also raises the issue of spatial resolution. Should the inhabitants of Palermo, for example, be referred to as Sicilian, Italian, Mediterranean, or European?

Of the many options for describing the geography of a sample using population labels, continental-scale summaries of geographic locations are among the most commonly used. Continental-scale population descriptors are problematic for two main reasons: the heterogeneity that exists within continents along nearly any dimension of interest, and the important fact that continent boundaries have no relevance for genetics studies. As examples, neither the classical divide of Asia and Europe in the Bosporus Strait nor separating Asia and Africa at the Suez Canal are meaningful indicators of genetic ancestry. The use of continents as a unit of analysis is arguably part of a larger intellectual tradition of mistakenly viewing continents as homogenous units (Lewis and Wigen, 1997).

Researchers may also face logistical challenges when trying to apply geographic population descriptors. They often have access to only a single self-reported location or one sampling location (like place of residence), but it may not be the location that is most relevant to address the study question (for example, birthplace). Or sometimes a geographic location is imputed from a group label, which inevitably misrepresents geographic origins. For example, for the purposes of carrying out a geographic analysis, a researcher might use the geographic center of France for all individuals labeled as French. In other cases, a geographic location will be intentionally coarse-grained to preserve privacy and hinder de-anonymizing individual-level data (e.g., the use of postal codes to represent geographic locations versus providing precise latitude and longitude). Whether such practices are problematic will depend on the type of analysis and the sensitivity it has to errors.

Finally, the fact that geography is often understood through the filter of geographical ancestry in many areas of genetics may lead to conceptual slippages. For example, in representations of the geography of human genetic variation, samples are often projected on maps according to the location of inferred ancestors rather than on the sampling location, such as placing the CEPH sample of Utah individuals (CEU) in the category of Central European ancestry, or the Gujaratis sampled in Houston (GIH) in South Asia in figures showing 1000 Genomes data (1000 Genomes Project Consortium, 2015). This slippage may be unimportant for questions related to understanding the genetic history of particular sets of peoples, but it is problematic in research in which geography is a proxy for environmental exposures. As another example, the People of the British Isles project describes the population genetic history of those people of the British Isles with recent ancestors from the British Isles,[2] leaving aside for future work understanding the histories of all individuals on the British Isles with recent ancestors from other parts of the world, such as immigrants from South Asia. Such approaches have implications for equity—by focusing on one geographic ancestry, a subset of participants is excluded from analyses. Another related limitation of geography as a population descriptor is its incompleteness. Individuals living within the same geographic area may be highly heterogeneous socially, ethnically, environmentally, and in terms of genetic ancestry. As with the use of genetic ancestry as a population descriptor, careful consideration of the intended uses of a geographic descriptor is essential in every genomics study.

Ethnicity

Ethnicity is often mentioned alongside race without clarifying the relationship between the two. Although the frequent expression *race and ethnicity* suggests they are separate concepts, it is not unusual for them to be treated as synonyms (or combined in the adjective *ethnoracial*) (Malinowska and Żuradzki, 2022). Their shared association with descent facilitates this elision, as does the not uncommon desire to find a substitute term for *race*.

Despite certain resemblances, the terms *ethnicity* and *race* have distinct conceptual histories and connotations. While the race notion was formed prior to the twentieth century, the idea of ethnicity was popularized in the early 1900s to capture differences between European-origin groups in the United States (Hattam, 2004). In this context, ethnicity was intended expressly to mean something other than race: linguistic, religious, and other cultural group markers as opposed to the physical traits that supposedly demarcated races.

Ethnicity then can be defined as a sociopolitical system for classifying human beings according to claims of shared heritage that are largely based on perceived cultural similarities (e.g., of language, dress, foodways, reli-

---

[2] University of Oxford. n.d. People of the British Isles: Population genetics and facial genetics. https://peopleofthebritishisles.web.ox.ac.uk/home (accessed October 19, 2022).

gion) (Cornell and Hartmann, 2007). Its similarity to race stems from the common claims to delineate descent-associated groups, but where racial boundaries have historically been closely tied to supposed biological traits, ethnic groupings are more tightly linked to perceived cultural practices, norms, values, and beliefs (Cornell and Hartmann, 2007).

The frequent conflation of race and ethnicity, however—in the United States and elsewhere (Wimmer, 2013)—means that ethnic groups may be racialized (e.g., ascribed ostensibly racial characteristics, for example in the case of Hispanics/Latinos in the United States), and racial groups can be ethnicized (e.g., Asians being ascribed broad cultural similarities).

The tendency for race and ethnicity—broadly understood as physical and cultural difference—to be intertwined when thinking about the groups that are seen as descending from shared roots means that they are perhaps more distinct in their abstract definitions than they are in everyday language and practice. It is useful, then, to draw a distinction between the separate logics at their core in order to clarify the concepts of difference that are in play when researchers design and assess genomics research.

The type of group that is recognized as an ethnicity varies widely. In the United States, descendants of voluntary immigrants are perhaps the most likely to be labeled as ethnic groups: hence Italian Americans, Korean Americans, and Cuban Americans, for example, are considered ethnic groups (Cornell and Hartmann, 2007). Although African Americans could also be said to constitute a culturally distinct ethnic group, their long and profound history of racialization[3] as black has tended to preclude recognition as an ethnic community (Clergé, 2019; Waters, 1990). However, as the African-descent population of the United States becomes increasingly diverse in terms of its migration background (Clergé, 2019; Hamilton, 2019), African Americans are likely to come to be better understood as an ethnic group distinct from, say, Haitian Americans or Nigerian Americans.

Another form of ethnicity that tends *not* to be recognized as such in the United States is indigeneity; instead, the language of *nations* and *tribes* endures to describe the wide variety of native North American groups that are heirs to distinct languages and traditions. The next section explores indigeneity in greater detail, but here the committee wishes to contrast the U.S. tendency to distinguish ethnicity from indigeneity, when outside the United States, *ethnicity* may often denote groups that are considered indigenous to a given territory. Worldwide, then, ethnicity is not limited to a product of migration.

The United States is also unusual for its official system of ethnoracial classification (OMB Statistical Directive 15), which recognizes only one

---

[3] Racialization is the process through which groups defined by attributes or characteristics such as skin color, customs, etc. come to be understood as distinct biological entities and human lineages (Hochman, 2019).

ethnicity today: Hispanic or Latino identification. Normally, official questions about ethnicity—notably, as they appear on national censuses—offer respondents a wide range of options from which to choose. The 2021 Canadian census, for example, instructs respondents to indicate as many "ethnic or cultural origins" as applicable and provides a link to a list of more than 500 examples.[4] This report does not adopt the OMB's equation of ethnicity with Hispanicity, but rather it uses the term to denote inclusive and comprehensive classification schema that recognize multiple ethnic groups.

One of the most common ways in which geneticists have incorporated ethnicity in their research is through the inclusion of linguistic information (Barbujani and Sokal, 1990; Cavalli-Sforza et al., 1988; Wang et al., 2007). As Cavalli-Sforza (1997) contended in his study of human genetic history:

> Most patterns found in the analysis of human living populations are likely to be consequences of demographic expansions, determined by technological developments affecting food availability, transportation, or military power. During such expansions, both genes and languages are spread to potentially vast areas. In principle, this tends to create a correlation between the respective evolutionary trees. The correlation is usually positive and often remarkably high. (p. 7719)

Linguistics thus often marks the migration of populations across geographic space, as language is something they "carry" with them. As is demonstrated by Western-Hemisphere societies in which such European languages as English and Spanish predominate even though large swathes of their populations trace their roots outside Europe, mother tongues do not necessarily mirror ancestral origins. The reach of language as a reflection of descent is therefore time sensitive, a factor that must be taken into account by researchers who wish to use linguistic data as a measure of ethnicity.

Linguistic patterns are also likely to deviate from other descent-associated population descriptors. But to the extent that a researcher may wish to capture an ethnic sense of belonging; gauge familiarity with the worldviews, norms, and values expressed through a particular language; or link exposure to particular ethnic practices or institutions, language may be of real use as a descent-associated population descriptor. In data collection from living individuals, information on language usage and fluency may be self-reported (or assessed by an external evaluation), whereas the genetic investigations of human evolutionary history that have effectively

---

[4] See Canada's long-form 2021 questionnaire at https://www.statcan.gc.ca/en/statistical-programs/instrument/3901_Q2_V6, and its Examples of Ethnic or Cultural Origins at https://www12.statcan.gc.ca/census-recensement/2021/ref/questionnaire/ancestry.cfm (both accessed December 13, 2022).

incorporated language data have tended to rely on classifications developed by linguistic experts (Tishkoff et al., 2009).

In summary, using ethnicity as a population descriptor has the advantage of offering myriad ways to capture it—and thus the challenge of selecting and justifying the choice from among many options. As is true of other descriptors considered in this report, it requires the researcher to reflect carefully and precisely on the mechanism they wish to explore and to collect the data that best measure the variable(s) they have in mind.

Indigeneity

The term *Indigenous* is generally applied to peoples who retain a historical link to precolonial societies in a given place or region (Martínez Cobo, 1987). Its definition is complex, however, and its use and meaning may differ between local contexts. Like ethnicity, indigeneity carries connotations of descent-associated cultural traditions, and in some places (including the United States), it has been translated into racial categories that emphasize physical traits and political status (Gartner et al., 2021). However, the concept of indigeneity is distinguished from these other population descriptors by its emphasis on the continuity of geographic location over time as well as shared culture, traditions, and other connections (Bello-Bravo, 2019).

The social salience of indigeneity varies a great deal across the globe. The recognition of indigeneity seems to be more common in regions and countries outside Europe that have been subjected to Europeans' relatively recent colonial expansions. Accordingly, the label *Indigenous* is rarely applied to populations within Europe itself—that is, the Sámi are the only Indigenous people recognized within the European Union (The Swedish Development Forum, 2018). Consistent with this observation, a study of censuses conducted around the world between 1995 and 2004 found that no European nation fielded a question on Indigenous or tribal status, compared to 67 percent of those in South America, where it was most frequent (Morning, 2008).

There are also striking differences in the terminology used to refer to Indigenous peoples around the world (Bartlett et al., 2007). Variants of the term "Indian" (e.g., *American Indian*, *indio*) continue to be widely used across the Americas to refer to Indigenous ancestries from the Western Hemisphere, in the biomedical literature as well as in popular parlance (Benedet et al., 2012; Egan et al., 2017; Goicoechea et al., 2001; Guardado-Estrada et al., 2009; Marca-Ysabel et al., 2021; Spangenberg et al., 2021). Indigenous peoples in Australia are often referred to as "aboriginal" (Malaspinas et al., 2016; Nasir et al., 2022; Rasmussen et al., 2011), whereas New Zealand is more specific in recognizing the Māori as Indigenous and distinguishing them from other Polynesian populations in the West Pacific, which are often referred to with geographic labels such as Tongan, Samoan, or Cook Islanders (Tätte et al., 2022; Umaefulam et al., 2022; Wang et al., 2022). In short, the nomenclature associated with indigeneity goes from very broad and homogenizing groupings—such as *native* or *Indian*—that primarily serve to distinguish them from the non-Indigenous, to much narrower, more geographically delimited ethnic identifiers such as Māori or Lenape (Peters, 2011). Depending on the granularity of these descriptors, genomics studies can have very different resolutions and interpretations, and, therefore, comparability to other studies.

In addition to its association with geographical rootedness over time, indigeneity often carries a connotation of "purity" or absence of admixture with non-Indigenous peoples. In such interpretations, indigeneity functions as a racial category, complete with the kind of references to blood quantum (as in *half-blood* or *full-blood*) that played an important role in the development of the race concept (Gartner et al., 2021). Today, American Indian/Alaska Native peoples in the United States often have to prove and substantiate their tribal enrollment status through blood quantum in order to qualify for health and other governmental benefits specified by treaty obligations (Spruhan, 2017).

Many countries have adopted (or inherited) classification systems that aim to discern different degrees of mixing between European and Indigenous populations during and since colonial times; the *castas* taxonomies of Spanish colonies in the Americas offer a prime example (Katzew, 2004; Moreno Navarro, 1973). This is especially evident in areas where admixture was believed to lead to the "whitening"—and ultimate disappearance—of Indigenous peoples, releasing their lands for European occupation (Wolfe, 2001).

Such is the case of the term *mestizo* (Spanish for admixed), which is used across Spanish-speaking Latin America, including in the biomedical and genetics literature (Silva-Zolezzi et al., 2009; Wang et al., 2008). In colonial times, *mestizo* was used to refer to the offspring of Spaniards with Indigenous partners, and over time it has been generalized to distinguish almost everyone who is not Indigenous (Rodriguez Mega, 2021). Thus, as with other group labels, *mestizo* is inaccurate because it socially homogenizes a genetically heterogeneous group of people.

The U.S. terms *American Indian* and *Alaska Native* are broadly used to describe the more than 574 federally recognized tribal nations (excluding the state-recognized or unrecognized tribes), each of which exists as a sovereign entity with its own distinct culture and language (NCAI, 2020). Tribal nations have final determination of who they designate as tribal members, sometimes determined through direct familial ties, descent, or through a minimum blood quantum value (U.S. Department of the Interior, n.d.). The terms *Hispanic* and *Latino* also amount to broad single descriptors applied to a heterogeneous and diverse group of populations with varying degrees of recent African, European, and Indigenous American genetic ancestries (Bryc et al., 2010, 2015). In Canada, the term *Métis* refers to individuals of mixed recent European (primarily French) and Indigenous genetic ancestry, distinguishing them from First Nations and Inuit Indigenous peoples (Bartlett et al., 2007).

In other regions of the world, such as North Africa, the Middle East, and Central Asia, there is not a generalized term that aims to distinguish Indigenous from admixed peoples. Despite the high degree of admixture among North Africans, primarily involving Indigenous North African ancestry, near Eastern Arab ancestry, and European ancestry, or across Asia between Turkic and Mongolian groups and earlier inhabitants, Indigenous ancestries tend to be described in the literature by either specific geographic terms (e.g., Maghrebi, Qatari) or specific ethnicities (e.g., Berber, Saharawi, Bedouin, Hazara, Azeri) (Botigué et al., 2013; Henn et al., 2012; Koshy et al., 2017; Rodriguez-Flores et al., 2016). In these regions where the degree of European ancestry is not a focal point for describing admixture, indigeneity is not perceived as distinct from or inconsistent with admixture. In self-identified Berber as well as Arab communities in North Africa, local populations are often described as mixtures of various Indigenous components (Arauna et al., 2017; Lucas-Sánchez et al., 2021).

Despite the variety of conceptual and terminological approaches to indigeneity found around the world, a common theme is that of the sensitivity of nomenclature and classification. This is not unique to indigeneity; other population descriptors raise similar issues. Yet labels of *Indigenous* clearly pose myriad difficulties. For one thing, the widely used term *Indian* for the original inhabitants of the Western Hemisphere is a well-known misnomer, even as it has been broadly used by both Indigenous and non-Indigenous Americans (Snipp and National Committee for Research on the 1980 Census, 1989; Snipp, 2002). In Australia, the term "aboriginal" has come under scrutiny for its association with a long and ongoing history of discrimination as well as controversial research practices (Kowal et al., 2012). And the categories meant to distinguish admixed populations from supposedly "pure" Indigenous ones are, as shown previously, overly broad and homogenizing.

These challenges and others make clear that researchers must employ population labels with great care, paying attention to their connotations (historical and contemporary), understanding the terms preferred by the groups in question, and whenever possible, engaging with the communities affected to arrive at descriptors that respect group self-understandings and self-identification. An example is the effort led by Māori researchers in biobanking and genetics research in New Zealand; they worked to incorporate Māori perspectives from the outset to provide a framework for global consideration of Indigenous knowledge in describing and engaging with local communities (Beaton et al., 2017; Kathlene et al., 2022).

Race

The concept of race has roots in the European project of settler-colonialism and slavery and emerged gradually over the sixteenth to nineteenth centuries (Keel, 2018; Mahmud, 1999). Race as it is understood today derives from historical and modern forms of racism and while racial thinking shares certain elements in common with other classification systems based on, say, religion or color, race differs in the specific configuration of assumptions made about the nature of human difference. Smedley and Smedley (2012) identify five ideological ingredients of the racial worldview as it developed in the United States:

1. All humans can be categorized into a universal set of self-evident, discrete, exclusive biological groups.
2. These groups are ranked hierarchically.
3. Surface-level traits used to demarcate races, such as skin color, reflect deeper, essential differences in cognitive, cultural, or moral attributes.
4. These attributes are heritable, such that essential differences remain stable over time.
5. These distinct groups exist in nature or are the product of divine creation.

These assumptions are not unique to the United States; they also characterize forms of racial classification that crystallized in other contexts of European settler-colonialism by the nineteenth century, such as in South America or Australia (Wolfe, 2016). Across these varied settings, race is fundamentally a sociopolitically constructed system for classifying and ranking human beings according to subjective beliefs about shared ancestry and innate biological similarities.

Race was integral to Enlightenment-era understandings of human nature and helped to resolve a contradiction reflected in two competing elements of political and social discourse (Fredrickson, 2002; Keel, 2018; Roberts, 2011). On the one hand, Western political theorists and actors championed the principles of liberty, equality, rights, and happiness. On the other hand, however, their societies were deeply enmeshed in colonialism and enslavement, which were enormously profitable for elites but the antithesis of democratic values. Theories of race resolved the contradiction between the discourse of liberty and the reality of slavery by inventing hierarchical taxonomies of fixed subdivisions, or types, of humankind, each with different capacities and natural stations in life. The supposedly superior and inferior races that Linnaeus and other early scientists described were not thought to possess the same rights, privileges, or even humanity—

thus seemingly justifying the freedom of some and the subjugation of others (Guyatt, 2016; Morgan, 1975; Wolfe, 2016).

The history of race, science, and society is important for contemporary genetics and genomics researchers to understand, because it illustrates that race emerged as a political project well before the development of population genetics or the evolutionary theory that sustains it. However, including that history here in sufficient detail is beyond the scope of this report and outside the committee's statement of task. For a deeper understanding of race and racism and their impacts on science and society, begin with the references in Box 1-1.

The social nature of race is especially evident in the United States, where it was not only embedded in early governing structures like the Constitution or naturalization law, but where racial categories have constantly evolved. The list of racial groups on the U.S. Census, for example, has changed nearly every decade since the first enumeration in 1790 (Figure 2-2), with categories like "mulatto," "Mexican," and "Hindu" appearing and disappearing (Lee, 1993; Prewitt, 2005). In the early twentieth century, Italians, Jews, and the Irish were popularly considered to be racial groups, distinct from the white majority with Northern European ancestry (Jacobson, 1998). There have been profound disagreements in both the demarcations between races and the meaning of race itself. These disagreements have never been only a battle of abstract ideas—or of scientific precision. Racial thinking emerges from historical and contemporary forms of racism and retains its force because of the way it buttresses political, economic, and social structures.

In addition to the dynamic nature of how race is conceptualized, race is also a complex population descriptor because it can be interpreted and measured in many ways. As sociologist Wendy Roth (2016) puts it, race is "multidimensional," and she identifies six broad dimensions of race:

1. "Racial identity" refers to an individual's self-identification;
2. "Racial self-classification" describes how an individual reports their race in formal settings with a limited menu of options, like on a census form;
3. "Observed race" is the race that observers ascribe to an individual, based on appearance or behavior;
4. "Reflected race" is what an individual believes others take them to be;
5. "Phenotype" corresponds to visible physical traits that are thought to be indicators of racial membership; and
6. "Racial ancestry" captures the racial identities ascribed to one's ancestors (as reported by family lore, for example, or inferred by genetic genealogy companies).

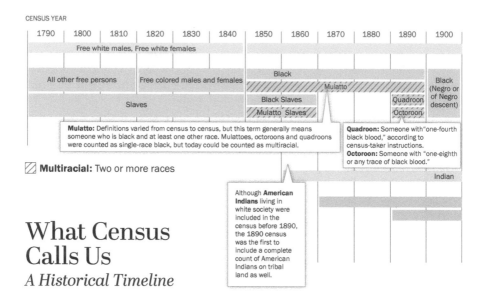

CENSUS YEAR

| 1790 | 1800 | 1810 | 1820 | 1830 | 1840 | 1850 | 1860 | 1870 | 1880 | 1890 | 1900 |

Free white males, Free white females

All other free persons | Free colored males and females

Black

Mulatto

Black (Negro or of Negro descent)

Slaves

Black Slaves

Mulatto Slaves

Quadroon

Octoroon

Mulatto: Definitions varied from census to census, but this term generally means someone who is black and at least one other race. Mulattoes, octoroons and quadroons were counted as single-race black, but today could be counted as multiracial.

Quadroon: Someone with "one-fourth black blood," according to census-taker instructions.
Octoroon: Someone with "one-eighth or any trace of black blood."

Indian

▨ **Multiracial:** Two or more races

Although **American Indians** living in white society were included in the census before 1890, the 1890 census was the first to include a complete count of American Indians on tribal land as well.

What Census Calls Us
A Historical Timeline

This graphic displays the different race, ethnicity and origin categories used in the U.S. decennial census, from the first one in 1790 to the latest count in 2020. The category names often changed from one decade to the next, in a reflection of current politics, science and public attitudes. For example, "colored" became "black," with "Negro" and "African American" added later. The term "Negro" was dropped for the 2020 census. Through 1950, census-takers commonly determined the race of the people they counted. From 1960 on, Americans could choose their own race. Starting in 2000, Americans could include themselves in more than one racial category. Before that, many multiracial people were counted in only one racial category.

FIGURE 2-2 U.S. Census race and ethnicity categories over time (1790–2020). SOURCE: Pew Research Center, https://www.pewresearch.org/wp-content/up-loads/2020/02/PH_15.06.11_MultiRacial-Timeline.pdf. Courtesy of Pew Research Center.

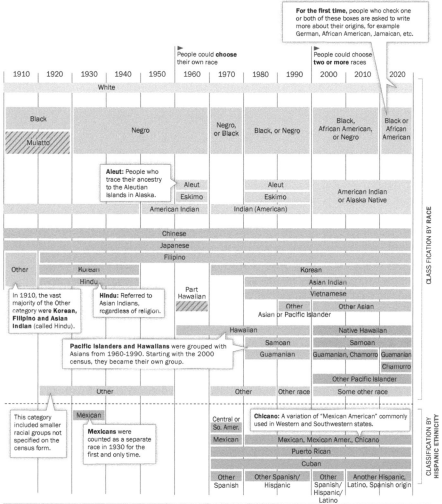

For the first time, people who check one or both of these boxes are asked to write more about their origins, for example German, African American, Jamaican, etc.

People could **choose** their own race

People could choose **two or more** races

| 1910 | 1920 | 1930 | 1940 | 1950 | 1960 | 1970 | 1980 | 1990 | 2000 | 2010 | 2020 |

White

Black

Mulatto

Negro

Negro, or Black

Black, or Negro

Black, African American, or Negro

Black or African American

Aleut: People who trace their ancestry to the Aleutian Islands in Alaska.

Aleut

Eskimo

American Indian

Aleut

Eskimo

Indian (American)

American Indian or Alaska Native

Chinese

Japanese

Filipino

Other

Korean

Hindu

Korean

Asian Indian

In 1910, the vast majority of the Other category were **Korean, Filipino and Asian Indian** (called Hindu).

Hindu: Referred to Asian Indians, regardless of religion.

Part Hawaiian

Vietnamese

Other

Asian or Pacific Islander

Other Asian

Hawaiian

Native Hawaiian

Pacific Islanders and Hawaiians were grouped with Asians from 1960-1990. Starting with the 2000 census, they became their own group.

Samoan

Guamanian

Samoan

Guamanian, Chamorro

Guamanian

Chamorro

Other Pacific Islander

Other

Other

Other race

Some other race

CLASSIFICATION BY **RACE**

This category included smaller racial groups not specified on the census form.

Mexican

Mexicans were counted as a separate race in 1930 for the first and only time.

Central or So. Amer.

Mexican

Chicano: A variation of "Mexican American" commonly used in Western and Southwestern states.

Mexican, Mexican Amer., Chicano

Puerto Rican

Cuban

Other Spanish

Other Spanish/ Hispanic

Other Spanish/ Hispanic/ Latino

Another Hispanic, Latino, Spanish origin

CLASSIFICATION BY **HISPANIC ETHNICITY**

PEW RESEARCH CENTER

As research on individuals' "contested identities" shows, these dimensions are not necessarily aligned with each other (Vargas and Kingsbury, 2016). An individual who self-identifies as Asian and white might check off "white" alone on a survey yet be perceived as Asian by an observer. In the rare cases where race is used as a proxy for the experience of racism in health disparities studies and its genetic contributions, researchers should carefully consider which dimension of racial identity is best suited to their study objective, be mindful of which dimension of race their data actually measures, and be transparent in specifying it.

As these dimensions of race suggest, it is also important to indicate the source of racial data: are the data based on individuals' self-reports of their racial identity? Or perhaps an external observers' impressions of their phenotype? Equally important is acknowledging the fluidity of racial identity, making it crucial to indicate the point in time at which the data were collected. Liebler et al. (2017) determined that nearly 10 million individuals changed their racial self-classification on the U.S. census between 2000 and 2010, making clear that race should not be presumed to be a stable personal characteristic over time. Andrew Penner and Aliya Saperstein show, moreover, that not only are such fluctuating racial categorizations true of observers' reports as well, but that these changes in racial identification—whether individually chosen or externally assessed—are associated with the social status of the individual whose race is being identified (Penner and Saperstein, 2018; Saperstein and Penner, 2012).

For all these reasons (and more—see Box 1-1 and Chapter 1), race makes for a poor proxy of human biological variation. However, it may be a useful population descriptor for researchers who wish to measure a consequential form of social status and affiliation, in the absence of other data (notably, the case where race may be a proxy for the experience of racism in health disparities studies, see Chapter 5). As W.E.B. Du Bois (1923) famously put it, "the black man is a person who must ride 'Jim Crow' in Georgia." This definition tells us that while race lacks the precision, rigor, stability, and objectivity one might hope for in a population descriptor, it is a social construct that speaks volumes about its time and place. Applied to any specific human being, however, it is a blunt instrument with which to infer individual social standing, economic status, or experiences of discrimination (Monk, 2022). For this reason, the committee urges researchers to think deeply about the specific experiences, characteristics, or outcomes they wish to investigate, and then consider searching for or constructing measures that capture these more directly and precisely than race ever can.

THE IMPORTANCE OF ENVIRONMENTAL FACTORS IN GENETICS AND GENOMICS RESEARCH

This final section of the chapter touches on three topics. First, the genome does not operate in a physiological vacuum. An organism's internal milieu and the external world it inhabits interact with the genome to affect phenotypic expression and variability (Alon, 2006). Second, to better understand the interplay of genes and the environment in humans, descent-associated population descriptors should frequently be accompanied by measures of the population's relevant environment(s) in genetics studies. Finally, researchers are increasing the understanding of environment effects on phenotypes through studies of the epigenome—the sum total of all chemical modifications that occur on the DNA sequence of the genome to modulate the activity of genes (Felsenfeld, 2015). The epigenome can thus be viewed as one liaison between the environment and the genome. Hence, it will be increasingly valuable to incorporate epigenetic measurements into studies of human genetic variation.

Genes, Environments, and their Interactions

It has long been recognized that phenotypes are the result of interplay between an individual's genome and their environment (Li et al., 2018; Seabrook and Avison, 2010; Strickberger, 1985). Breeders and farmers have used this knowledge for centuries to select for and breed crops and domestic animals with desirable traits. Genetics studies have shown us that this interplay is complex, dynamic, and often hard to untangle. A gene's expression depends on a range of factors from an organism's internal physiologic state to signals received about the immediate external milieu, as well as on the stage of the cell cycle and the state of the epigenome (Boyce et al., 2020). Importantly, the genome interacts with the environment throughout an individual's lifetime to form an aggregate phenotype.

Some of the earliest genetics studies in the fruit fly *Drosophila*, corn, and the bread mold *Neurospora* examined the effects of the external environment such as temperature, light, and nutrition, respectively, on the occurrence of mutations (genetic variants) (Strickberger, 1985). Other studies, including in humans, examined the effects of the internal environment as measured by age and sex (Strickberger, 1985). This body of literature suggested two new insights: (1) some genotypes exhibit differential expression depending on the environment (a gene–environment interaction) (Gibson, 2008; Smith and Kruglyak, 2008), and (2) relatives share not only genes but also an environment, called the shared environment, which leads to a correlation of genetic backgrounds with environments (Mayhew and Meyre, 2017). Thus, phenotypic similarity of two individuals depends on their genetic variation profiles (genotypes), their shared and unique environments, as well as the resulting interactions between each individual's genome and their environment (see the effects on stature in Jelenkovic et al., 2016).

So, what might be the consequence of ignoring the environment? When the environmental effects vary, then failing to take them into account is at best incomplete and more likely misleading. This might arise in two ways. First, the environment can vary independent of genes, as most genetics studies assume. Not studying the environment in this case means that the analysis is incomplete, and further, generalizing the effects of the genetics that were uncovered to new environmental settings is problematic and can be error prone. Second, the environment covaries with genetics so that interpreting the results of phenotypic similarity in terms of genetics alone would simply be misleading and can overemphasize its effects (Mayhew and Meyre, 2017).

Defining the Environment

Settling on a definition of the *environment* is tricky, because it is contextual, varies among scientific disciplines, and necessarily groups highly diverse concepts under one umbrella term. As Robette (2022) observes,

> One might wonder what effects the use of the term environment without epistemological scrutiny has on the construction of sociological objects. In the additive polygenic model, the environment is anything that is not genetic. In the context of epidemiology, the environment refers mainly to risk factors (diet, pollution, etc.). For sociogenomicists, the environment seems synonymous with the social. The use of the term without conceptual work thus leads to the grouping of highly diverse processes under the same term. (pp. 198-199)

For any given study, a researcher has to identify which environmental factors to examine and how to measure them accurately, as with any descent-associated population descriptors.

For any given trait, only a limited number of environmental factors are likely at play, some of which can be gleaned from the epidemiologic literature. In the absence of directly measuring environmental factors, epidemiologic and genetics studies sometimes use race or ethnicity as a proxy for measures such as cultural beliefs or shared environment (Benmarhnia et al., 2021; Duello et al., 2021; Martinez et al., 2022).

Social context, an attribute of the environment, influences behavior and interacts dynamically with biology, including genetics, throughout the life course to affect human health (Glass and McAtee, 2006). The social context or social environment can be defined as the society and physical surroundings and conditions in which a person lives, works, and interacts with others. It can be measured in a variety of ways, capturing multiple dimensions

(Boardman et al., 2012; Duncan and Kawachi, 2018; Williams et al., 2019). It can be objective or perceived/self-reported and can vary in spatial scale depending on the boundaries set by geography and/or the researcher (Diez Roux and Mair, 2010; Duncan and Kawachi, 2018). Heuristically, the social environment can be classified into two broad categories, which are not necessarily mutually exclusive and may interact with each other:

1. Social conditions: examples include social support, social networks, income inequality, deprivation and poverty, education, social capital, segregation, discrimination, demographic composition, and violence.
2. Built or physical environment: examples include land use, green spaces, pollution, traffic noise, and population density.

Structural racism is a system of oppression that shapes the conditions and resources of the environment, such as those listed in the two categories above. Researchers are starting to measure structural racism using a combination of variables at the state and Metropolitan Statistical Area levels (Hardeman et al., 2022; Homan et al., 2021; Krieger, 2021). The concentration of racialized and ethnic groups in the United States is unevenly distributed owing to sociopolitical processes such as segregation and poverty (Williams et al., 2019); therefore, to avoid biologizing race and ethnicity, it is especially important to directly quantify the environment when conducting research aimed at understanding phenotypes that result from both genetic and environmental effects. This is necessary because genetic variation and environmental effects can be correlated or interact. Correlation occurs when genotypes or presumed ancestries are not randomly distributed across environments (e.g., ancestries of children exposed to lead-based paint in their homes), and interaction happens when genetic effects depend on the environment (e.g., phenylketonuria occurs only with phenylalanine in the diet). Thus, ancestry-specific or ancestry-enriched markers may show an excess with the developmental growth outcomes measured from lead exposure, but these are hardly the biological etiologic factors geneticists wish to discover. Some genetics studies can correct this effect in part using genetic markers, but the etiologic factor is lead. Yet in both examples, recognition of the environmental agent is central to understanding the outcomes and phenotypes that result from both genetic and environmental effects. Furthermore, for example, residential segregation and community demographic composition are considered in multilevel analysis to capture social exposures that may be embodied and affect an individual's biology (e.g., psychosocial stress associated with living in a poor neighborhood may lead to hypertension) (Arcaya and Schnake-Mahl, 2017; Kramer and Hogue, 2009; Parks, 2016; Williams and Collins, 2001).

Much of the evidence on the association between environmental factors and health draws on studies centered on spatially defined geographic areas. Some of the spatially defined areas are viewed as proxies for neighborhood. However, neighborhood boundaries are often inferred from administrative areas (e.g., census-defined geographic areas such as tracts, block groups, and zip codes) rather than neighborhoods defined more in terms of social boundaries or even ecological boundaries. Other spatially defined boundaries are also possible based on proximity to the individual (e.g., the density of violence), and persons often cross boundaries in their daily lives, bringing into play multiple types of environmental influences.

The preceding discussion emphasizes that although researchers can qualitatively and quantitatively measure some aspects of the environment related to individual research participants, this cannot, with today's knowledge, be complete. Unlike the genome, which is large yet finite and can be studied completely (at some level of resolution), an exhaustive characterization of environmental effects is not feasible. It is difficult to determine the critical period, the dose-response, or the specific environmental factor affecting the human genome. In addition, most environmental factors are correlated with each other as they may be determined by the same upstream cause, e.g., structural racism. These limitations represent key challenges for the interpretation of genetics and genomics studies but compel us to begin to make meaningful strides toward defining the roles of selected and plausible common and unique environments in the traits studied, though admittedly, this is a much harder task for some phenotypes than for others. Consequently, there may be merit to studies of the epigenome that can capture some of the cellular consequences of environmental effects even when the specific environment is unknown.

Epigenetics as Environmental Sensors

Environmental exposures can change gene expression and a consequent phenotype. For example, a remarkable study seeking the molecular causes of thalidomide embryopathy demonstrated that thalidomide phenocopies Mendelian genetic syndromes (Donovan et al., 2018). Starting with a previous observation that genetic mutations in the transcription factor *SALL4* led to Duane Radial Ray syndrome and Holt-Oram syndrome, the authors showed that thalidomide directly degrades the SALL4 protein. There are other compelling examples, such as induced nicotinamide adenine dinucleotide (NAD) deficiency in the offspring of mice. Restricting the NAD precursors tryptophan and vitamin B3 in the maternal diet during pregnancy led to an increased frequency of miscarriages and congenital abnormalities in their offspring (Cuny et al., 2020). Interestingly, recessive homozygous variants in *HAAO* or *KYNU*, two genes of the NAD synthesis pathway, cause similar phenotypes in humans and mice, whereas a single copy of these variants that does not lead to an abnormal phenotype alone can be made to do so when combined with maternal diet-mediated NAD deficiency. The molecular basis and the developmental pathways involved are well defined, as they are for the etiology of congenital scoliosis (Sparrow et al., 2012). Taken together, these and other studies imply that (1) phenotype similarity between two individuals can arise from genes only, environments only, genes in one and the environment in the other, or from the interactions between genes and the environment in the same individual, and (2) despite the different proximal causes, the distal molecular causes of the effects of environmental perturbations and those of genetic variants can converge on the same molecular process and the same molecules, at some rate-limiting step (Chakravarti and Turner, 2016).

The question is how genetic and environmental effects—two different proximal causes—can mediate the same outcome. The answer often involves the epigenome. There are two major paths to these changes. In the first, the genome sequence is chemically modified by DNA methylation, which alters the expression of genes (Allis et al., 2015). This process is both genetically programmed and affected by external environment factors, such as diet (Dolinoy, 2008). In the second, the expression of each gene is exquisitely controlled by RNA and protein molecules such that its transcription into RNA and translation into protein is monitored and that information is fed back to regulate the gene's level and timing of expression (Davidson, 2010). This regulatory machinery, also epigenetic, involves chromatin, transcription factors, and enhancer sequences that are bound by the transcription factors (Allis et al., 2015). Both types of epigenetic machinery are important determinants of phenotype expression (Chakravarti and Turner, 2016). This molecular machinery can today be defined for each human cell type and tissue, and its variation studied in differential traits (e.g., normotensives versus hypertensives). Consequently, a person's epigenome appears to be functioning as a possible sensor of the environment in which they reside.

An important unanswered question that arises from the above discussion is the time period over which the effects of an exposure can be detected in the epigenome. Some epigenetic modifications, such as parent-of-origin-specific genomic imprinting, are genetically programmed and have lifelong effects on gene and organismal physiology. Others, such as the effects of dietary manipulations, particularly those that affect DNA methylation, are short term, though when they occur early in development can have long-term phenotypic effects (Weyrich et al., 2018). In general, however, the timing, maintenance, or erasure of epigenetic effects on the human genome and phenotype is a largely unexplored area of study.

Epigenetics holds some promise for understanding the consequences of the role of some environments over the life course, especially windows of vulnerability such as childhood that may have long-term consequences for traits decades later in life (Shanahan and Hofer, 2011). This has given rise to the evolving area of social epigenetics (Evans et al., 2021; Martin et al., 2022). However, there needs to be further research on the causal relationship between the external and internal pathways and how these lead to phenotypic change.

Quantifying Environments at the Individual Level

Environmental variables used in research studies can be qualitative or quantitative. There is merit to variables that are quantitative or metrical and show a monotonic relationship with a phenotype of interest (e.g., blood pressure) or disease risk (e.g., hypertension-induced target organ damage). Whenever feasible, these should be measured at the individual research participant level similar to how genotypes are measured. However, this is a highly challenging endeavor. The exposures relevant to different phenotypes may be during development or in years past and, thus, almost impossible to measure, although there may be an epigenetic imprint of such exposures. Even when an exposure is proximal, such as in the survivors of the atomic bombings in Hiroshima and Nagasaki, individual-level radiation exposure was very challenging to quantify because it depended on distance from the blast site, whether the individual was inside or outside, and the type of dwelling in which they resided, among other factors (NRC, 1991). Thus, in many investigations, the only plausible contrast may be between cases and controls, rather than exposed versus unexposed, with no resolution at the level of the individual.

The interest on the part of such funding agencies as the National Institute of Environmental Health Sciences to further develop "exposome" science, preferably inclusive of the "socioexposome," is laudatory.[5] The interest in obtaining multiscale measures of the geospatial environment for large-scale population studies is of great benefit to genetics (Cui et al., 2022). Like the Human Genome Project, which had a staged approach to developing higher resolution and more accurate maps of the human genome, similar efforts in developing individual-level and dynamic exposome measures are necessary to understand the full spectrum of genes, environments, and their interactions, both in individuals and in populations.

---

[5] https://www.niehs.nih.gov/research/supported/exposure/bio/index.cfm (accessed January 3, 2023).

REFERENCES

1000 Genomes Project Consortium. 2015. A global reference for human genetic variation. *Nature* 526:68-74.

Allis, C. D., M. L. Caparros, T. Jenuwein, and D. Reinberg. 2015. *Epigenetics.* 2nd ed. Cold Spring Harbor, NY: Cold Spring Harbor Laboratory Press.

Alon, U. 2006. *An introduction to systems biology: Design principles of biological circuits.* 1st ed. London: CRC Press.

Arauna, L. R., J. Mendoza-Revilla, A. Mas-Sandoval, H. Izaabel, A. Bekada, S. Benhamamouch, K. Fadhlaoui-Zid, P. Zalloua, G. Hellenthal, and D. Comas. 2017. Recent historical migrations have shaped the gene pool of Arabs and Berbers in North Africa. *Molecular Biology and Evolution* 34(2):318-329.

Arcaya, M. C., and A. Schnake-Mahl. 2017. Health in the segregated city. In *The dream revisited.* New York: NYU Furman Center.

Barbujani, G., and R. R. Sokal. 1990. Zones of sharp genetic change in Europe are also linguistic boundaries. *Proceedings of the National Academy of Sciences* 87(5):1816-1819.

Bartlett, J. G., L. Madariaga-Vignudo, J. D. O'Neil, and H. V. Kuhnlein. 2007. Identifying indigenous peoples for health research in a global context: A review of perspectives and challenges. *International Journal of Circumpolar Health* 66(4):287-370.

Beaton, A., M. Hudson, M. Milne, R. V. Port, K. Russell, B. Smith, V. Toki, L. Uerata, P. Wilcox, K. Bartholomew, and H. Wihongi. 2017. Engaging Māori in biobanking and genomic research: A model for biobanks to guide culturally informed governance, operational, and community engagement activities. *Genetics and Medicine* 19(3):345-351.

Bello-Bravo, J. 2019. When is indigeneity: Closing a legal and sociocultural gap in a contested domestic/international term. *AlterNative: An International Journal of Indigenous Peoples* 15(2):111-120.

Benedet, A. L., C. F. Moraes, E. F. Camargos, L. F. Oliveira, V. C. Souza, T. C. Lins, A. D. Henriques, D. G. Carmo, W. Machado-Silva, C. N. Araújo, C. Córdova, R. W. Pereira, and O. T. Nóbrega. 2012. Amerindian genetic ancestry protects against Alzheimer's disease. *Dementia and Geriatric Cognitive Disorders* 33(5):311-317.

Benmarhnia, T., A. Hajat, and J. S. Kaufman. 2021. Inferential challenges when assessing racial/ethnic health disparities in environmental research. *Environmental Health* 20(1):7.

Boardman, J. D., E. Roettger, B. W. Domingue, M. B. McQueen, B. C. Haberstick, and K. M. Harris. 2012. Gene-environment interactions related to body mass: School policies and social context as environmental moderators. *Journal of Theoretical Politics* 24(3):370-388.

Botigué, L. R., B. M. Henn, S. Gravel, B. K. Maples, C. R. Gignoux, E. Corona, G. Atzmon, E. Burns, H. Ostrer, C. Flores, J. Bertranpetit, D. Comas, and C. D. Bustamante. 2013. Gene flow from North Africa contributes to differential human genetic diversity in southern Europe. *Proceedings of the National Academy of Sciences* 110(29):11791-11796.

Boyce, W. T., M. B. Sokolowski, and G. E. Robinson. 2020. Genes and environments, development and time. *Proceedings of the National Academy of Sciences* 117(38):23235-23241.

Bryc, K., C. Velez, T. Karafet, A. Moreno-Estrada, A. Reynolds, A. Auton, M. Hammer, C. D. Bustamante, and H. Ostrer. 2010. Colloquium paper: Genome-wide patterns of population structure and admixture among Hispanic/Latino populations. *Proceedings of the National Academy of Sciences* 107(Suppl 2):8954-8961.

Bryc, K., E. Y. Durand, J. M. Macpherson, D. Reich, and J. L. Mountain. 2015. The genetic ancestry of African Americans, Latinos, and European Americans across the United States. *American Journal of Human Genetics* 96(1):37-53.

Cavalli-Sforza, L. L. 1997. Genes, peoples, and languages. *Proceedings of the National Academy of Sciences* 94(15):7719-7724.

Cavalli-Sforza, L. L., A. Piazza, P. Menozzi, and J. Mountain. 1988. Reconstruction of human evolution: Bringing together genetic, archaeological, and linguistic data. *Proceedings of the National Academy of Sciences* 85(16):6002-6006.

Chakraborty, R., and K. M. Weiss. 1986. Frequencies of complex diseases in hybrid populations. *American Journal of Physical Anthropology* 70(4):489-503.

Chakravarti, A., and T. N. Turner. 2016. Revealing rate-limiting steps in complex disease biology: The crucial importance of studying rare, extreme-phenotype families. *Bioessays* 38(6):578-586.

Chandra, K. 2012. *Constructivist theories of ethnic politics.* Oxford University Press.

Clergé, O. 2019. *The new noir: Race, identity, and diaspora in black suburbia.* Berkeley, CA: University of California Press.

Coop, G. 2023. Genetic similarity versus genetic ancestry groups as sample descriptors in human genetics. *arXiv* (preprint).

Coop Lab. 2017a. *Our vast, shared family tree.* https://gcbias.org/2017/11/20/our-vast-shared-family-tree/ (accessed November 7, 2022).

Coop Lab. 2017b. *Where did your genetic ancestors come from?* https://gcbias.org/2017/12/19/1628/ (accessed October 20, 2022).

Cornell, S., and D. Hartmann. 2007. *Ethnicity and race: Making identities in a changing world.* Thousand Oaks, CA: Pine Forks Press.

Cui, Y., K. M. Eccles, R. K. Kwok, B. R. Joubert, K. P. Messier, and D. M. Balshaw. 2022. Integrating multiscale geospatial environmental data into large population health studies: Challenges and opportunities. *Toxics* 10(7):403.

Cuny, H., M. Rapadas, J. Gereis, E. M. M. A. Martin, R. B. Kirk, H. Shi, and S. L. Dunwoodie. 2020. NAD deficiency due to environmental factors or gene-environment interactions causes congenital malformations and miscarriage in mice. *Proceedings of the National Academy of Sciences* 117(7):3738-3747.

Davidson, E. H. 2010. Emerging properties of animal gene regulatory networks. *Nature* 468:911-920.

Diez Roux, A. V., and C. Mair. 2010. Neighborhoods and health. *Annals of the New York Academy of Sciences* 1186:125-145.

Dolinoy, D. C. 2008. The agouti mouse model: An epigenetic biosensor for nutritional and environmental alterations on the fetal epigenome. *Nutrition Review* 66(Suppl 1):S7-S11.

Donnelly, K. P. 1983. The probability that related individuals share some section of genome identical by descent. *Theoretical Population Biology* 23(1):34-63.

Donovan, K. A., J. An, R. P. Nowak, J. C. Yuan, E. C. Fink, B. C. Berry, B. L. Ebert, and E. S. Fischer. 2018. Thalidomide promotes degradation of SALL4, a transcription factor implicated in Duane-radial ray syndrome. *eLife* 7:e38430.

Du Bois, W. E. B. 1923. The superior race (an essay). *The Smart Set: A Magazine of Cleverness* 70(4):55-60.

Duello, T. M., S. Rivedal, C. Wickland, and A. Weller. 2021. Race and genetics versus 'race' in genetics: A systematic review of the use of African ancestry in genetic studies. *Evolution, Medicine, and Public Health* 9(1):232-245.

Duncan, D. T., and I. Kawachi. 2018. *Neighborhoods and health.* 2nd ed. Oxford, UK: Oxford University Press.

Egan, K. J., H. Campos Santos, F. Beijamini, N. E. Duarte, A. R. V. R. Horimoto, T. P. Taporoski, H. Vallada, A. B. Negrão, J. E. Krieger, M. Pedrazzoli, K. L. Knutson, A. C. Pereira, and M. von Schantz. 2017. Amerindian (but not African or European) ancestry is significantly associated with diurnal preference within an admixed Brazilian population. *Chronobiology International* 34(2):269-272.

Evans, L., M. Engelman, A. Mikulas, and K. Malecki. 2021. How are social determinants of health integrated into epigenetic research? A systematic review. *Social Science in Medicine* 273:113738.

Falush, D., M. Stephens, and J. K. Pritchard. 2003. Inference of population structure using multilocus genotype data: Linked loci and correlated allele frequencies. *Genetics* 164(4):1567-1587.

Felsenfeld, G. 2015. A brief history of epigenetics. In *Epigenetics*. 2nd ed., edited by C. D. Allis, M. L. Caparros, T. Jenuwein, and D. Reinberg. Cold Spring Harbor: Cold Spring Harbor Laboratory Press. Pp. 1-10.

Frederickson, G. M. 2002. *Racism: A short history*. Princeton, NJ: Princeton University Press.

Freedman, M. L., C. A. Haiman, N. Patterson, G. J. McDonald, A. Tandon, A. Waliszewska, K. Penney, R. G. Steen, K. Ardlie, E. M. John, I. Oakley-Girvan, A. S. Whittemore, K. A. Cooney, S. A. Ingles, D. Altshuler, B. E. Henderson, and D. Reich. 2006. Admixture mapping identifies 8q24 as a prostate cancer risk locus in African-American men. *Proceedings of the National Academy of Sciences* 103(38):14068-14073.

Fujimura, J. H., and R. Rajagopalan. 2011. Different differences: The use of 'genetic ancestry' versus race in biomedical human genetic research. *Social Studies of Science* 41(1):5-30.

Gartner, D. R., R. E. Wilbur, and M. L. McCoy. 2021. "American Indian" as a racial category in public health: Implications for communities and practice. *American Journal of Public Health* 111(11):1969-1975.

Gibson, G. 2008. The environmental contribution to gene expression profiles. *Nature Reviews Genetics* 9(8):575-581.

Glass, T. A., and M. J. McAtee. 2006. Behavioral science at the crossroads in public health: Extending horizons, envisioning the future. *Social Science & Medicine* 62(7):1650-1671.

Goicoechea, A. S., F. R. Carnese, C. Dejean, S. A. Avena, T. A. Weimer, M. H. L. P. Franco, S. M. Callegari-Jacques, A. C. Estalote, M. L. Simões, M. Palatnik, and F. M. Salzano. 2001. Genetic relationships between Amerindian populations of Argentina. *American Journal of Physical Anthropology* 115(2):133-143.

Guardado-Estrada, M., E. Juarez-Torres, I. Medina-Martinez, A. Wegier, A. Macías, G. Gomez, F. Cruz-Talonia, E. Roman-Bassaure, D. Piñero, S. Kofman-Alfaro, and J. Berumen. 2009. A great diversity of Amerindian mitochondrial DNA ancestry is present in the Mexican mestizo population. *Journal of Human Genetics* 54:695-705.

Guyatt, N. 2016. *Bind us apart: How enlightened Americans invented racial segregation*. Oxford University Press.

Haak, W., I. Lazaridis, N. Patterson, N. Rohland, S. Mallick, B. Llamas, G. Brandt, S. Nordenfelt, E. Harney, K. Stewardson, Q. Fu, A. Mittnik, E. Bánffy, C. Economou, M. Francken, S. Friederich, R. G. Pena, F. Hallgren, V. Khartanovich, A. Khokhlov, M. Kunst, P. Kuznetsov, H. Meller, O. Mochalov, V. Moiseyev, N. Nicklisch, S. L. Pichler, R. Risch, M. A. Rojo Guerra, C. Roth, A. Szécsényi-Nagy, J. Wahl, M. Meyer, J. Krause, D. Brown, D. Anthony, A. Cooper, K. W. Alt, and D. Reich. 2015. Massive migration from the steppe was a source for Indo-European languages in Europe. *Nature* 522(7555):207-211.

Hamilton, T. G. 2019. *Immigration and the remaking of black America*. New York: Russell Sage Foundation.

Hannaford, I. 1996. *Race: The history of an idea in the west*. Washington, DC: Woodrow Wilson Center Press.

Hardeman, R. R., P. A. Homan, T. Chantarat, B. A. Davis, and T. H. Brown. 2022. Improving the measurement of structural racism to achieve antiracist health policy. *Health Affairs* 41(2):179-186.

Hattam, V. 2004. Ethnicity: An American genealogy. In *Not just black and white: Historical and contemporary perspectives on immigration, race, and ethnicity in the United States*. Edited by N. Foner and G. M. Fredrickson. New York: Russell Sage Foundation. Pp. 42-60.

Henn, B. M., L. R. Botigué, S. Gravel, W. Wang, A. Brisbin, J. K. Byrnes, K. Fadhlaoui-Zid, P. A. Zalloua, A. Moreno-Estrada, J. Bertranpetit, C. D. Bustamante, and D. Comas. 2012. Genomic ancestry of North Africans supports back-to-Africa migrations. *PLoS Genetics* 8(1):e1002397.

Hochman, A. 2019. Racialization: A defense of the concept. *Ethnic and Racial Studies* 42(8):1245-1262.

Homan, P., T. H. Brown, and B. King. 2021. Structural intersectionality as a new direction for health disparities research. *Journal of Health and Social Behavior* 62(3):350-370.

Hollinger, A. 1998. National culture and communities of descent. *Reviews in American History* 26(1):312-328.

Hudson, R. R. 1990. Gene genealogies and the coalescent process. *Oxford Surveys in Evolutionary Biology* 7(1):44.

Jacobson, M. F. 1998. *Whiteness of a different color: European immigrants and the alchemy of race.* Cambridge, MA: Harvard University Press.

Jelenkovic, A., R. Sund, Y.-M. Hur, Y. Yokoyama, J. v. B. Hjelmborg, S. Möller, C. Honda, P. K. E. Magnusson, N. L. Pedersen, S. Ooki, S. Aaltonen, M. A. Stazi, C. Fagnani, C. D'Ippolito, D. L. Freitas, J. A. Maia, F. Ji, F. Ning, Z. Pang, E. Rebato, A. Busjahn, C. Kandler, K. J. Saudino, K. L. Jang, W. Cozen, A. E. Hwang, T. M. Mack, W. Gao, C. Yu, L. Li, R. P. Corley, B. M. Huibregtse, C. A. Derom, R. F. Vlietinck, R. J. F. Loos, K. Heikkilä, J. Wardle, C. H. Llewellyn, A. Fisher, T. A. McAdams, T. C. Eley, A. M. Gregory, M. He, X. Ding, M. Bjerregaard-Andersen, H. Beck-Nielsen, M. Sodemann, A. D. Tarnoki, D. L. Tarnoki, A. Knafo-Noam, D. Mankuta, L. Abramson, S. A. Burt, K. L. Klump, J. L. Silberg, L. J. Eaves, H. H. Maes, R. F. Krueger, M. McGue, S. Pahlen, M. Gatz, D. A. Butler, M. Bartels, T. C. E. M. van Beijsterveldt, J. M. Craig, R. Saffery, L. Dubois, M. Boivin, M. Brendgen, G. Dionne, F. Vitaro, N. G. Martin, S. E. Medland, G. W. Montgomery, G. E. Swan, R. Krasnow, P. Tynelius, P. Lichtenstein, C. M. A. Haworth, R. Plomin, G. Bayasgalan, D. Narandalai, K. P. Harden, E. M. Tucker-Drob, T. Spector, M. Mangino, G. Lachance, L. A. Baker, C. Tuvblad, G. E. Duncan, D. Buchwald, G. Willemsen, A. Skytthe, K. O. Kyvik, K. Christensen, S. Y. Öncel, F. Aliev, F. Rasmussen, J. H. Goldberg, T. I. A. Sørensen, D. I. Boomsma, J. Kaprio, and K. Silventoinen. 2016. Genetic and environmental influences on height from infancy to early adulthood: An individual-based pooled analysis of 45 twin cohorts. *Scientific Reports* 6(1):28496.

Kathlene, L., D. Munshi, P. Kurian, and S. L. Morrison. 2022. Cultures in the laboratory: Mapping similarities and differences between Māori and non-Māori in engaging with gene-editing technologies in Aotearoa, New Zealand. *Humanities and Social Sciences Communications* 9(100).

Katzew, I. 2004. *Casta painting: Images of race in eighteenth-century Mexico.* New Haven, CT: Yale University Press.

Keel, T. 2018. *Divine variations: How Christian thought became racial science.* 1st ed. Stanford, CA: Stanford University Press.

Kelleher, J., A. M. Etheridge, and G. McVean. 2016. Efficient coalescent simulation and genealogical analysis for large sample sizes. *PLoS Computational Biology* 12(5):e1004842.

Koshy, R., A. Ranawat, and V. Scaria. 2017. Al mena: A comprehensive resource of human genetic variants integrating genomes and exomes from Arab, Middle Eastern and north African populations. *Journal of Human Genetics* 62(10):889-894.

Kowal, E., G. Pearson, C. S. Peacock, S. E. Jamieson, and J. M. Blackwell. 2012. Genetic research and aboriginal and Torres Strait islander Australians. *Journal of Bioethical Inquiry* 9(4):419-432.

Kramer, M. R., and C. R. Hogue. 2009. Is segregation bad for your health? *Epidemiologic Reviews* 31(1):178-194.

Krieger, N. 2021. Structural racism, health inequities, and the two-edged sword of data: Structural problems require structural solutions. *Frontiers in Public Health* 9.

Lee, S. M. 1993. Racial classifications in the U.S. census: 1890–1990. *Ethnic and Racial Studies* 16(1):75-94.

Lewis, M. W., and K. E. Wigen. 1997. *The myth of continents: A critique of metageography.* Berkeley, CA: University of California Press.

Li, X., T. Guo, Q. Mu, X. Li, and J. Yu. 2018. Genomic and environmental determinants and their interplay underlying phenotypic plasticity. *Proceedings of the National Academy of Sciences* 115(26):6679-6684.

Liebler, C. A., S. R. Porter, L. E. Fernandez, J. M. Noon, and S. R. Ennis. 2017. America's churning races: Race and ethnic response changes between census 2000 and the 2010 census. *Demography* 54:259-284.

Lipson, M., P.-R. Loh, A. Levin, D. Reich, N. Patterson, and B. Berger. 2013. Efficient moment-based inference of admixture parameters and sources of gene flow. *Molecular Biology and Evolution* 30(8):1788-1802.

Lucas-Sánchez, M., J. M. Serradell, and D. Comas. 2021. Population history of north Africa based on modern and ancient genomes. *Human Molecular Genetics* 30(R1):R17-R23.

Mahmud, T. 1999. Colonialism and modern constructions of race: A preliminary inquiry. *University of Miami Law Review* 53:1219-1249.

Malaspinas, A. S., M. C. Westaway, C. Muller, V. C. Sousa, O. Lao, I. Alves, A. Bergström, G. Athanasiadis, J. Y. Cheng, J. E. Crawford, T. H. Heupink, E. Macholdt, S. Peischl, S. Rasmussen, S. Schiffels, S. Subramanian, J. L. Wright, A. Albrechtsen, C. Barbieri, I. Dupanloup, A. Eriksson, A. Margaryan, I. Moltke, I. Pugach, T. S. Korneliussen, I. P. Levkivskyi, J. V. Moreno-Mayar, S. Ni, F. Racimo, M. Sikora, Y. Xue, F. A. Aghakhanian, N. Brucato, S. Brunak, P. F. Campos, W. Clark, S. Ellingvåg, G. Fourmile, P. Gerbault, D. Injie, G. Koki, M. Leavesley, B. Logan, A. Lynch, E. A. Matisoo-Smith, P. J. McAllister, A. J. Mentzer, M. Metspalu, A. B. Migliano, L. Murgha, M. E. Phipps, W. Pomat, D. Reynolds, F. X. Ricaut, P. Siba, M. G. Thomas, T. Wales, C. M. Wall, S. J. Oppenheimer, C. Tyler-Smith, R. Durbin, J. Dortch, A. Manica, M. H. Schierup, R. A. Foley, M. M. Lahr, C. Bowern, J. D. Wall, T. Mailund, M. Stoneking, R. Nielsen, M. S. Sandhu, L. Excoffier, D. M. Lambert, and E. Willerslev. 2016. A genomic history of aboriginal Australia. *Nature* 538(7624):207-214.

Malinowska, J., and T. Żuradzki. 2022. Reductionist methodology and the ambiguity of the categories of race and ethnicity in biomedical research: An exploratory study of recent evidence. *Medicine, Health Care and Philosophy* 26(3):1-14.

Marca-Ysabel, M. V., F. Rajabli, M. Cornejo-Olivas, P. G. Whitehead, N. K. Hofmann, M. Z. Illanes Manrique, D. M. Veliz Otani, A. K. Milla Neyra, S. Castro Suarez, M. Meza Vega, L. D. Adams, P. R. Mena, I. Rosario, M. L. Cuccaro, J. M. Vance, G. W. Beecham, N. Custodio, R. Montesinos, P. E. Mazzetti Soler, and M. A. Pericak-Vance. 2021. Dissecting the role of Amerindian genetic ancestry and the ApoE ε4 allele on Alzheimer disease in an admixed Peruvian population. *Neurobiology and Aging* 101:298.e211-298.e215.

Martin, C. L., L. Ghastine, E. K. Lodge, R. Dhingra, and C. K. Ward-Caviness. 2022. Understanding health inequalities through the lens of social epigenetics. *Annual Review of Public Health* 43:235-254.

Martinez, R. A. M., N. Andrabi, A. N. Goodwin, R. E. Wilbur, N. R. Smith, and P. N. Zivich. 2022. Conceptualization, operationalization, and utilization of race and ethnicity in major epidemiology journals, 1995–2018: A systematic review. *American Journal of Epidemiology* 192(3):483-496.

Martínez Cobo, J. R. 1987. Study of the problem of discrimination against indigenous populations: Conclusions, proposals and recommendation. Vol. V. New York: United Nations.

Mathieson, I., and A. Scally. 2020. What is ancestry? *PLoS Genetics* 16(3):e1008624.

Mayhew, A. J., and D. Meyre. 2017. Assessing the heritability of complex traits in humans: Methodological challenges and opportunities. *Current Genomics* 18(4):332-340.

Monk, E. P. 2022. Inequality without groups: Contemporary theories of categories, intersectional typicality, and the disaggregation of difference. *Sociological Theory* 40(1):3–27.

Moreno Navarro, I. 1973. *Los "cuadros del mestizaje americano": Estudio antropológico del mestizaje.* Madrid, Spain: Ediciones Jose Porrua Turanzas.

Morgan, E. S. 1975. *American slavery, American freedom: The ordeal of colonial Virginia.* New York: W.W. Norton.

Morning, A. 2008. Ethnic classification in global perspective: A cross-national survey of the 2000 census round. *Population Research and Policy Review* 27:239-272.

Morning, A., and M. Maneri. 2022. *An ugly word: Rethinking race in Italy and the United States.* New York: Russell Sage Foundation.

Nasir, B. F., R. Vinayagam, and K. Rae. 2022. "It's what makes us unique": Indigenous Australian perspectives on genetics research to improve comorbid mental and chronic disease outcomes. *Current Medical Research and Opinion* 38(7):1219-1228.

NCAI (National Congress of American Indians). 2020. *Tribal nations and the United States: An introduction.* Washington, DC: National Congress of American Indians.

NRC (National Research Council). 1991. *The children of atomic bomb survivors: A genetic study.* Edited by J. V. Neel and W. J. Schull. Washington, DC: National Academy Press.

Parks, T. 2016. How racism, segregation drive health disparities. In *Patient support & advocacy.* Chicago, IL: American Medical Association.

Patterson, N., P. Moorjani, Y. Luo, S. Mallick, N. Rohland, Y. Zhan, T. Genschoreck, T. Webster, and D. Reich. 2012. Ancient admixture in human history. *Genetics* 192(3):1065-1093.

Penner, A. M., and A. Saperstein. 2008. How social status shapes race. *Proceedings of the National Academy of Sciences* 105:19628-19630.

Peters, E. J. 2011. Still invisible: Enumeration of indigenous peoples in census questionnaires internationally. *Aboriginal Policy Studies* 1(2):68-100.

Pickrell, J. K., and J. K. Pritchard. 2012. Inference of population splits and mixtures from genome-wide allele frequency data. *PLoS Genetics* 8(11):e1002967.

Prewitt, K. 2005. Racial classification in America: Where do we go from here? *Daedalus* 134(1):5-17.

Pritchard, J. K., M. Stephens, and P. Donnelly. 2000. Inference of population structure using multilocus genotype data. *Genetics* 155(2):945-959.

Rasmussen, M., X. Guo, Y. Wang, K. E. Lohmueller, S. Rasmussen, A. Albrechtsen, L. Skotte, S. Lindgreen, M. Metspalu, T. Jombart, T. Kivisild, W. Zhai, A. Eriksson, A. Manica, L. Orlando, F. M. De La Vega, S. Tridico, E. Metspalu, K. Nielsen, M. C. Ávila-Arcos, J. V. Moreno-Mayar, C. Muller, J. Dortch, M. T. Gilbert, O. Lund, A. Wesolowska, M. Karmin, L. A. Weinert, B. Wang, J. Li, S. Tai, F. Xiao, T. Hanihara, G. van Driem, A. R. Jha, F. X. Ricaut, P. de Knijff, A. B. Migliano, I. Gallego Romero, K. Kristiansen, D. M. Lambert, S. Brunak, P. Forster, B. Brinkmann, O. Nehlich, M. Bunce, M. Richards, R. Gupta, C. D. Bustamante, A. Krogh, R. A. Foley, M. M. Lahr, F. Balloux, T. Sicheritz-Pontén, R. Villems, R. Nielsen, J. Wang, and E. Willerslev. 2011. An Aboriginal Australian genome reveals separate human dispersals into Asia. *Science* 334(6052):94-98.

Reich, D. 2018. *Who we are and how we got here: Ancient DNA and the new science of the human past.* Oxford University Press.

Reich, D., A. L. Price, and N. Patterson. 2008. Principal component analysis of genetic data. *Nature Genetics* 40(5):491-492.

Roberts, D. 2011. *Fatal invention: How science, politics, and big business re-create race in the twenty-first century.* New York: The New Press.

Robette, N. 2022. The dead ends of sociogenomics. *Population* 77(2):181-216.

Rodriguez-Flores, J. L., K. Fakhro, F. Agosto-Perez, M. D. Ramstetter, L. Arbiza, T. L. Vincent, A. Robay, J. A. Malek, K. Suhre, L. Chouchane, R. Badii, A. Al-Nabet Al-Marri, C. Abi Khalil, M. Zirie, A. Jayyousi, J. Salit, A. Keinan, A. G. Clark, R. G. Crystal, and J. G. Mezey. 2016. Indigenous Arabs are descendants of the earliest split from ancient Eurasian populations. *Genome Research* 26(2):151-162.

Rodriguez Mega, E. 2021. How the mixed-race mestizo myth warped science in Latin America. *Nature* 600(7889):374-378.

Rohde, D. L. T., S. Olson, and J. T. Chang. 2004. Modelling the recent common ancestry of all living humans. *Nature* 431(7008):562-566.

Rosenberg, N. A. 2021. A population-genetic perspective on the similarities and differences among worldwide human populations. *Human Biology* 92(3):135-152.

Rosenberg, N. A., J. K. Pritchard, J. L. Weber, H. M. Cann, K. K. Kidd, L. A. Zhivotovsky, and M. W. Feldman. 2002. Genetic structure of human populations. *Science* 298(5602):2381-2385.

Roth, W. D. 2016. The multiple dimensions of race. *Ethnic and Racial Studies* 39:1310-1338.

Saperstein, A., and A. M. Penner. 2012. Racial fluidity and inequality in the United States. *American Journal of Sociology* 118:676-727.

Schaefer, N. K., B. Shapiro, and R. E. Green. 2021. An ancestral recombination graph of human, Neanderthal, and Denisovan genomes. *Scientific Advances* 7(29):eabc0776.

Seabrook, J. A., and W. R. Avison. 2010. Genotype–environment interaction and sociology: Contributions and complexities. *Social Science & Medicine* 70(9):1277-1284.

Shanahan, M. J., and S. M. Hofer. 2011. Molecular genetics, aging, and well-being: Sensitive period, accumulation, and pathway models. In *Handbook of aging and the social sciences*. 7th ed., edited by L. K. George. Elsevier. Pp. 135-147.

Silva-Zolezzi, I., A. Hidalgo-Miranda, J. Estrada-Gil, J. C. Fernandez-Lopez, L. Uribe-Figueroa, A. Contreras, E. Balam-Ortiz, L. del Bosque-Plata, D. Velazquez-Fernandez, C. Lara, R. Goya, E. Hernandez-Lemus, C. Davila, E. Barrientos, S. March, and G. Jimenez-Sanchez. 2009. Analysis of genomic diversity in Mexican mestizo populations to develop genomic medicine in Mexico. *Proceedings of the National Academy of Sciences* 106(21):8611-8616.

Smedley, A., and B. D. Smedley. 2012. *Race in North America: Origin and evolution of a worldview*. 4th ed. Oxfordshire, UK: Routledge.

Smith, E. N., and L. Kruglyak. 2008. Gene–environment interaction in yeast gene expression. *PLoS Biology* 6(4):e83.

Snipp, C. M. 2002. American Indians: Clues to the future of other racial groups. In *The new race question: How the census counts multiracial individuals*, edited by J. Perlmann and M. C. Waters. New York and Annandale-on-Hudson, NY: Russell Sage Foundation and Levy Economics Institute of Bard College. Pp. 189-214.

Snipp, C. M., and National Committee for Research on the 1980 Census. 1989. *American Indians: The first of this land*. New York: Russell Sage Foundation.

Spangenberg, L., M. I. Fariello, D. Arce, G. Illanes, G. Greif, J.-Y. Shin, S. K. Yoo, J. S. Seo, C. Robello, C. Kim, J. Novembre, M. Sans, and H. Naya. 2021. Indigenous ancestry and admixture in the Uruguayan population. *Frontiers of Genetics* 12:733195.

Sparrow, D. B., G. Chapman, A. J. Smith, M. Z. Mattar, J. Major, V. C. O'Reilly, Y. Saga, E. Zackai, J. Dormans, A. Benjamin, L. McGregor, R. Kageyama, K. Kusumi, and S. Dunmoodie. 2012. A mechanism for gene-environment interaction in the etiology of congenital scoliosis. *Cell* 149(2):295-306.

Spruhan, P. 2017. CDIB: The role of the certificate of degree of Indian blood in defining Native American legal identity. *American Indian Law Journal* 6:169.

Strickberger, M. W. 1985. *Genetics*. 3rd ed. New York: Macmillan.

The Swedish Development Forum. 2018. *Europe's only recognized indigenous peoples live in Sweden*. https://fuf.se/en/magasin/europas-enda-erkanda-urfolk-bor-i-sverigre/ (accessed December 13, 2022).

Tätte, K., E. Metspalu, H. Post, L. Palencia-Madrid, J. R. Luis, M. Reidla, E. Tamm, A. M. Ilumäe, M. M. de Pancorbo, R. Garcia-Bertrand, M. Metspalu, and R. J. Herrera. 2022. Genetic characterization of populations in the Marquesas Archipelago in the context of the Austronesian expansion. *Scientific Reports* 12:5312.

Thompson, E. A. 2013. Identity by descent: Variation in meiosis, across genomes, and in populations. *Genetics* 194(2):301-326.

Tishkoff, S. A., F. A. Reed, F. R. Friedlaender, C. Ehret, A. Ranciaro, A. Froment, J. B. Hirbo, A. A. Awomoyi, J. M. Bodo, O. Doumbo, M. Ibrahim, A. T. Juma, M. J. Kotze, G. Lema, J. H. Moore, H. Mortensen, T. B. Nyambo, S. A. Omar, K. Powell, G. S. Pretorius, M. W. Smith, M. A. Thera, C. Wambebe, J. L. Weber, and S. M. Williams. 2009. The genetic structure and history of Africans and African Americans. *Science* 324(5930):1035-1044.

Umaefulam, V., T. Kleissen, and C. Barnabe. 2022. The representation of indigenous peoples in chronic disease clinical trials in Australia, Canada, New Zealand, and the United States. *Clinical Trials* 19(1):22-32.

U.S. Department of the Interior. n.d. *Tribal enrollment process.* https://www.doi.gov/tribes/enrollment#main-content (accessed December 14, 2022).

Vargas, N., and J. Kingsbury. 2016. Racial identity contestation: Mapping and measuring racial boundaries. *Sociology Compass* 10(8):718-729.

Wang, K., M. Cadzow, M. Bixley, M. P. Leask, M. E. Merriman, Q. Yang, Z. Li, R. Takei, A. Phipps-Green, T. J. Major, R. Topless, N. Dalbeth, F. King, R. Murphy, L. K. Stamp, J. Zoysa, Z. Wang, Y. Shi, and T. R. Merriman. 2022. A Polynesian-specific copy number variant encompassing the MICA gene associates with gout. *Human Molecular Genetics* 31(21):3757-3768.

Wang, S., C. M. Lewis, Jr., M. Jakobsson, S. Ramachandran, N. Ray, G. Bedoya, W. Rojas, M. V. Parra, J. A. Molina, C. Gallo, G. Mazzotti, G. Poletti, K. Hill, A. M. Hurtado, D. Labuda, W. Klitz, R. Barrantes, M. C. Bortolini, F. M. Salzano, M. L. Petzl-Erler, L. T. Tsuneto, E. Llop, F. Rothhammer, L. Excoffier, M. W. Feldman, N. A. Rosenberg, and A. Ruiz-Linares. 2007. Genetic variation and population structure in Native Americans. *PLoS Genetics* 3(11):e185.

Wang, S., N. Ray, W. Rojas, M. V. Parra, G. Bedoya, C. Gallo, G. Poletti, G. Mazzotti, K. Hill, A. M. Hurtado, B. Camrena, H. Nicolini, W. Klitz, R. Barrantes, J. A. Molina, N. B. Freimer, M. C. Bortolini, F. M. Salzano, M. L. Petzl-Erler, L. T. Tsuneto, J. E. Dipierri, E. L. Alfaro, G. Bailliet, N. O. Bianchi, E. Llop, F. Rothhammer, L. Excoffier, and A. Ruiz-Linares. 2008. Geographic patterns of genome admixture in Latin American mestizos. *PLoS Genetics* 4(3):e1000037.

Waters, M. C. 1990. *Ethnic options: Choosing identities in America.* Berkeley, CA: University of California Press.

Weyrich, A., D. Lenz, and J. Fickel. 2018. Environmental change-dependent inherited epigenetic response. *Genes* 10(4).

Williams, D. R., and C. Collins. 2001. Racial residential segregation: A fundamental cause of racial disparities in health. *Public Health Reports* 116(5):404-416.

Williams, D. R., J. A. Lawrence, and B. A. Davis. 2019. Racism and health: Evidence and needed research. *Annual Review of Public Health* 40:105-125.

Wimmer, A. 2013. *Ethnic boundary making: Institutions, power, networks.* Oxford, UK: Oxford University Press.

Wiuf, C., and J. Hein. 1999. Recombination as a point process along sequences. *Theoretical Population Biology* 55(3):248-259.

Wohns, A. W., Y. Wong, B. Jeffery, A. Akbari, S. Mallick, R. Pinhasi, N. Patterson, D. Reich, J. Kelleher, and G. McVean. 2022. A unified genealogy of modern and ancient genomes. *Science* 375(6583):eabi8264.

Wolfe, P. 2001. Land, labor, and difference: Elementary structures of race. *American Historical Review* 106(3):866-905.

Wolfe, P. 2016. *Traces of history: Elementary structures of race.* London: Verso Books.

SECTION II

RECOMMENDATIONS

SECTION II OVERVIEW

Section I set the stage for an imperative to transform both the conceptualization and use of population descriptors and the design of genetics and genomics studies. To that end, the recommendations offered in Section II are embedded within a multidimensional framework that provides a holistic approach to fostering and sustaining trustworthy (e.g., ethically and empirically sound) genetics and genomics research. For research findings to be trustworthy, they must be generated with validity and accuracy and under a commitment to using that research to advance the interests of the participants and provide benefits to broader society. In doing so, both the research and researcher become trustworthy. Therefore, the committee's recommendations span the genetics and genomics research ecosystem, recognizing the importance of various parties in facilitating systemic change in the field.

Section II comprises four chapters that provide a road map for an evolution of this research ecosystem. Researchers will be the ones to lead transformation of the field, influenced and supported by a variety of relevant parties. Thus, for the committee's recommendations to be successful, they must be grounded in key ethical and empirical principles that drive the trustworthiness of the research and build trust among all interested parties.

Chapter 3 presents a set of guiding principles that undergird the committee's recommendations. Chapter 4 provides recommendations on some overarching concerns that will have to be addressed to achieve sustained change in genetics and genomics practice and research. These items are dispelling typological thinking, engaging with communities of study participants, and integrating measurements of environmental factors in genomics research, whenever feasible. Chapter 5 offers detailed guidance and best practices to researchers concerning the use of population descriptors organized by type of genomics study. Chapter 6 focuses on implementation and accountability strategies for the relevant parties who support, influence, and communicate the work of the researchers (see Figure II-1 for a representation of the framework).

Researchers in human genetics and genomics have often struggled with a lack of clear, specific guidance. The recommendations and best practices offered in this section are, therefore, intended to operationalize the guiding principles with specific practices and procedures.

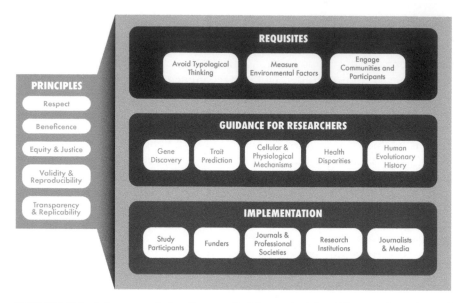

FIGURE II-1 A framework for change. Guiding principles (Chapter 3) undergird the subsequent recommendations, which fall into three categories: (1) requisites for transforming the use of population descriptors in human genomics research (Chapter 4), guidance for researchers conducting different types of genomics studies (Chapter 5), and implementation through various relevant parties to support researchers and promote change throughout the genomics research ecosystem (Chapter 6).

3

Guiding Principles

INTRODUCTION

The committee identified guiding principles intended to foster the highest ethical and empirical practices and to support trustworthy research to inform its recommendations. For scientific research to be trustworthy, it must be both ethically conducted and empirically valid (Beskow et al., 2021; Emanuel et al., 2000; Goering et al., 2008; NASEM, 2019); both aspects of trustworthiness reinforce each other. Indeed, as discussed in Chapters 1 and 2, the history of racialization and typological thinking about differences between human groups in genetics research produced unethical and invalid findings, which hindered the advancement of the science. The guiding principles discussed here aim to achieve these requirements of trustworthy research. Each recommendation in this report is motivated by at least one guiding principle and reflects commitments necessary from the scientific enterprise. In creating its recommendations and best practices, the committee has identified a range of studies and research contexts in which each would be applied. However, the research enterprise is dynamic, and it is impractical for this report to fully capture the range of possible use cases in future genetics and genomics research as technologies and perspectives change. Thus, the guiding principles provide a foundation and common vocabulary for interested parties to engage in future decision making for contexts that may not be addressed directly in this report.

The guiding principles outlined here address the ethical responsibilities of *respect*, *beneficence*, *equity*, and *justice*, as well as scientific standards of *validity*, *reproducibility*, *transparency*, and *replicability*. These principles together operate to build trust among researchers and the many relevant parties in the genomics research ecosystem. It is especially important to foster trust between researchers and study participants and with the general public (Beskow et al., 2021; Faure et al., 2021). By identifying these principles, the committee emphasizes ethical integrity and scientific best practices as foundational to the selection of population descriptors in human genetics and genomics research.

PRINCIPLES

Respect

Respect for individual and community preferences, norms, and values should inform approaches when determining population descriptors. Respect begins with the recognition that a person has the right to make decisions as an autonomous individual and is deserving of dignity (Lee, 2021). Acknowledging the important role of communities, the committee extends this principle to groups who have a stake in how they are characterized in genetics research. This principle of respect requires protecting the autonomy of individuals and communities in determining what data are collected and how data are characterized (Lee, 2021). For example, individuals and groups may prefer descriptors that reflect multiple and/or situationally specific identities. Respectful research requires engaging, understanding, and acting upon the perspectives, preferences, and lived experiences of individuals and communities (Goering et al., 2008; Lee, 2021). Respect should also address the desire among participants for nondisclosure of data and/or the possibility of an exit from studies (Beskow et al., 2021; Emanuel, et al., 2000). Trustworthiness of research depends on investigators demonstrating respect toward participants throughout the life course of a study, including study design, informed consent, managing samples, protecting private information, data safety monitoring, and dissemination (Beskow et al., 2021). Researchers and research institutions should explore strategies that can promote trustworthiness through collaboration and accountability mechanisms (see the section "Community Engagement" in Chapter 4).

Beneficence

Trustworthy and equitable science requires that research produces benefit for individuals, communities, and the public as well as promotes human dignity, although such benefits may not be immediate nor be tangible to the participant (Beskow et al., 2021; Emanuel et al., 2000). The principle of beneficence calls on researchers to assess how the selection of population descriptors may generate not only potential good but also potential harm. Fulfilling goals of beneficence requires consideration of the needs and interests of all relevant parties, including researchers, participants, communities, and the public at large (Claw et al., 2018; Lee, 2021). When considering the use of population descriptors, researchers have an obligation to use labels and methods that benefit individual participants and communities. Researchers must also avoid potential negative effects on groups, such as stigma, discrimination and exacerbation of racial and ethnic inequities, reinforcement of hierarchical and typological thinking, and inequitable distribution of benefits (Beskow et al., 2021; de Vries et al., 2012; Emanuel et al., 2000; Martin et al., 2022).

Equity and Justice[1]

Decisions about population descriptors should recognize the structural inequities in society, the histories of exploitation and abuse of politically marginalized groups participating in genetics research, and the effect and potential harm that research and the labels used will have on these groups. A commitment to justice and the goal of equity requires that researchers avoid reproducing hierarchical thinking embedded in the historical use of classification systems such as race in science. This commitment requires addressing whom researchers choose to study (sampling biases) and confronting the power imbalances in science, which have contributed to the lack of participation of historically marginalized groups (Martin et al., 2022; Mills and Rahal, 2020) and the disrespect of those who participate. Embedded within these commitments is a responsibility to ensure representative sampling wherever possible to answer specific research questions or achieve particular research goals.

A commitment to equity and justice, though, should be more than assessing representation in research participation; it should include addressing inequities in the scientific workforce and who is conducting research on whom, and their effects on the use of population descriptors in genetics research. Researchers should strive toward engaging communities early in the research process and to consider historical, political, and societal biases that may inform their descriptions. Researchers should avoid procedures that privilege particular viewpoints at the exclusion of those who have been historically marginalized and disempowered (Goering et al., 2012). In addition, a commitment to equity and justice requires an assessment of whether and how the selection and use of population descriptors will

---

[1] Equity "recognizes that each person has different circumstances and allocates the exact resources and opportunities needed to reach an equal outcome. Equity is a solution for addressing imbalanced social systems" (GWU, 2020). "Justice, or social justice, is the view that everyone deserves to enjoy the same economic, political, and social rights, regardless of race, socioeconomic status, gender, and other characteristics" (Begg, 2021).

produce equitable benefits and avoid reinforcing existing inequities or introducing new ones.

Validity and Reproducibility

Fulfilling the principle of validity requires judicious evaluation of research objectives, the use of resources, and potential risks and benefits of research. A study is valid if it is designed to yield reproducible data (NASEM, 2019), whereas studies that are poorly designed to answer research questions are scientifically invalid and unethical (Emanuel et al., 2000; NASEM, 2019). Researchers should be intentional in selecting population descriptors that will answer specific research questions. This will require assessing the appropriateness and purpose of including population descriptors for the type of study being conducted. Assessment of the validity of the use of population descriptors as well as the risks and benefits associated with the research should include the expertise of the communities involved (Claw et al., 2018). In addition, the principle of validity requires that study design and decision making on population descriptors enable reproducibility by independent researchers. For example, providing detailed definitions and descriptions of methodologies for selecting and applying population descriptors will support reproducibility of study findings across studies and the potential for accurately understanding study results.

Transparency and Replicability[2]

The principle of transparency includes the obligation to provide clear rationale for the selection and use of population descriptors and to explain decision-making processes in an open and accessible manner. This includes articulation of the conceptual assumptions and operational considerations that lead to the adoption of population descriptors. For example, procedures for achieving relative "homogeneity" in a data set or procedures of "binning" that combine data should be clearly described, including a rationale of why they are necessary. Such transparency is critical for rigor and replicability (NASEM, 2019). Articulation of methodological logic in a comprehensible manner can further empirical validation. In addition, participants in research should reasonably expect that researchers will communicate research goals and processes (Claw et al., 2018) and explain the selection of population descriptors used to describe them. Thus, adhering to the principle of transparency supports the principle of respect of individuals

---

[2] Replicability refers to obtaining consistent results across studies, as compared to reproducibility, which refers to obtaining consistent results from the same data set (NASEM, 2019).

and communities and their ability to assert autonomy and informed decision making about participation in research.

SYNERGY AMONG AND TENSION
BETWEEN GUIDING PRINCIPLES

These principles reflect values and goals that are overlapping, intertwined, and mutually reinforcing. All of the principles aim at a unified goal of engaging in scientifically valid and trustworthy research. Researchers should aim to achieve affinity among the principles. Nevertheless, tension between principles may arise when researchers prioritize competing interests. For example, group preferences for population descriptors may be in conflict with goals of reproducibility in which researchers use alternative descriptors to maximize data aggregation or harmonization (Lee et al., 2019). In such cases, researchers should make explicit their rationale for selecting specific population descriptors and assess how these decisions affect principles of responsible research and their potential effect on trustworthiness and equity. Ultimate decisions about the use of population descriptors may vary depending on the specific context of the research, responsiveness to community preferences, and evolving best practices over time. This concept will be explored further in Chapter 5.

The committee encourages all relevant parties, including researchers, institutions, funders, professional organizations, journals, media, and communities, to assess and engage in the discussion of how practices contribute to synergies among, and tensions between, guiding principles. The committee underscores the importance of collaboration when resolving competing interests. Power imbalances inherent in research, and research institutions, and the potential vulnerability of individuals and groups enrolled in research create challenges for equitable partnership and can undermine the trustworthiness of science (Faure et al., 2021; Parker and Kingori, 2016; Powers and Faden, 2019). Researchers should employ these guiding principles and explore strategies, such as community engagement, to support shared decision making about population descriptors.

REFERENCES

Begg, R. 2021. *There's equality, equity...And then there's justice.* https://news.asante.org/theres-equality-equity-and-then-theres-justice/ (accessed November 14, 2022).

Beskow, L. M., S. M. Fullerton, and W. Burke. 2021. Ethical issues in genetic epidemiology. In *Ethics and epidemiology.* 3rd ed., edited by S. S. Coughlin and A. Dawson. Oxford, UK: Oxford University Press.

Claw, K. G., M. Z. Anderson, R. L. Begay, K. S. Tsosie, K. Fox, N. A. Garrison, and Summer internship for Indigenous peoples in Genomics (SING) Consortium. 2018. A framework for enhancing ethical genomic research with Indigenous communities. *Nature Communications* 9:2957.

de Vries, J., M. Jallow, T. N. Williams, D. Kwiatkowski, M. Parker, and R. Fitzpatrick. 2012. Investigating the potential for ethnic group harm in collaborative genomics research in Africa: Is ethnic stigmatisation likely? *Social Science and Medicine* 75(8):1400-1407.

Emanuel, E. J., D. Wendler, and C. Grady. 2000. What makes clinical research ethical? *JAMA* 283(20):2701-2711.

Faure, M. C., N. S. Munung, N. A. B. Ntusi, B. Pratt, and J. de Vries. 2021. Mapping experiences and perspectives of equity in international health collaborations: A scoping review. *International Journal for Equity in Health* 20:28.

Goering, S., S. Holland, and K. Fryer-Edwards. 2008. Transforming genetic research practices with marginalized communities: A case for responsive justice. *Hastings Center Report* 38(2):43-53.

GWU (George Washington University). 2020. *Equity vs. equality: What's the difference?* https://onlinepublichealth.gwu.edu/resources/equity-vs-equality/ (accessed December 6, 2022).

Lee, S. S.-J. 2021. The ethics of consent in a shifting genomic ecosystem. *Annual Review of Biomedical Data Science* 4(1):145-164.

Lee, S. S.-J., S. M. Fullerton, A. Saperstein, and J. K. Shim. 2019. Ethics of inclusion: Cultivate trust in precision medicine. *Science* 364(6444):941-942.

Martin, A. R., R. E. Stroud II, T. Abebe, D. Akena, M. Alemayehu, L. Atwoli, S. B. Chapman, K. Flowers, B. Gelaye, S. Gichuru, S. M. Kariuki, S. Kinyanjui, K. J. Korte, N. Koen, K. C. Koenen, C. Newton, A. M. Olivares, S. Pollock, K. Post, I. Singh, D. J. Stein, S. Teferra, Z. Zingela, and L. B. Chibnik. 2022. Increasing diversity in genomics requires investment in equitable partnerships and capacity building. *Nature Genetics* 54(6):740-745.

Mills, M. C., and C. Rahal. 2020. The GWAS diversity monitor tracks diversity by disease in real time. *Nature Genetics* 52:242-243.

NASEM (National Academies of Sciences, Engineering, and Medicine). 2019. *Reproducibility and replicability in science.* Washington, DC: The National Academies Press.

Parker, M., and P. Kingori. 2016. Good and bad research collaborations: Researchers' views on science and ethics in global health research. *PLoS ONE* 11(10):e0163579.

Powers, M., and R. Faden. 2019. *Structural injustice: Power, advantage, and human rights.* Oxford, UK: Oxford University Press.

4

Requisites for Sustained Change

INTRODUCTION

The work of the committee has highlighted the need to attend to some overarching and long-standing issues that, if not more deliberately and fully addressed, will continue to impede progress in genetics and genomics research. The three topics of focus in this chapter—typological thinking, environmental factors, and community engagement—are not an exhaustive list and are not new, but the committee believes addressing them will be paramount to the long-term success of the best practices and implementation of recommendations in Chapters 5 and 6. In recent years, there has been increasing attention to environmental factors and community engagement in genetics research broadly (Green et al., 2020). Researchers in the field, as well as many others, however, have largely overlooked typological thinking, arguably the crux of the matter with regard to the use of descent-associated population descriptors. The consequences of failing to intentionally confront these topics are grave. Recognizing this, the committee has prioritized addressing typological thinking, environmental factors, and community engagement in its proposed framework for transforming the use of population descriptors in genetics and genomics research. The committee trusts that this will accelerate the expansion of current efforts in these critical areas and stimulate the development of new ones.

For each of the topics in this chapter, the committee indicates the guiding principles pertaining to the respective recommendations. These recommendations complement those in Chapter 5, and together they position researchers to lead the transformation of not only how population descriptors are conceptualized and used, but also how genetics and genomics research is implemented and interpreted. The recommendations in Chapter 6 are intended to provide the support system that researchers will need to facilitate this outcome.

TYPOLOGICAL THINKING

Erroneous categorical assumptions are scientifically and ethically detrimental, particularly when applied to studies of human history, identity, variation, and traits and diseases (Lee et al., 2008; Shim et al., 2014; Weiss and Lambert, 2014). There is a pervasive misconception and belief that humans can be grouped into discrete innate categories (Jorde and Wooding, 2004). The illusion of discontinuity between racialized groups has supported a history of typological and hierarchical thinking, which both classify individuals by type—ignoring variation—and rank people by status (for full definitions see Appendix B). These modes of thinking often spill over to other descent-associated population descriptors such as ethnicity and ancestry (Byeon et al., 2021; Fang et al., 2019). The structure of human genetic variation, though, is the result of human population movement and mixing and so is more related to geography than to any racial or ethnic classification (see the section "Features of Human Genome Variation" in Chapter 1) (Jorde and Wooding, 2004; Lewontin, 1972; Manica et al., 2005).

In particular, describing geography with continental-scale labels, such as continental ancestry, can reinforce typological thinking. These labels can bolster the disproven view that the human species can naturally be divided into a small number of groups, akin to races, that are genetically homogeneous within each (Romualdi et al., 2002). Assumptions of homogeneity at the continental level reinforce the myth of original "pure" populations and buttress the belief in a racial hierarchy. A common and long-standing example of typological categories is Blumenbach's hierarchical taxonomy (Marks, 1995; Painter, 2010), including the term *Caucasian*, a problematic term which is still frequently used in science and society (Popejoy, 2021). Moreover, the influence of Linnaeus' system of human classification can still be seen today in the categories used in the U.S. Census (Harawa and Ford, 2009). In providing the following conclusions and three recommendations, the committee intends to draw attention to pervasive aspects of typological thinking and especially problematic terminology. Terms that imply a biological classification of race should not be used. This is not simply a matter of replacing some terms with other, more palatable terms. The objective of the committee was not to provide an improved nomenclature or vocabulary but to challenge misconceptions and push the dialogue forward. Anyone working in this area must think carefully and make judgments with clear rationale as to which population descriptors (or classification schemes) to use, which labels to use, and why. The question of which descriptors to use is nuanced and addressed in subsequent recommendations in this report. Guidance and tools for making these selections are provided in Chapter 5.

Conclusions and Recommendations

Conclusion 4-1. Race is neither useful nor scientifically valid as a measure of the structure of human genetic variation.

Conclusion 4-2. Using socially constructed groupings indiscriminately in human genetics research can be harmful. Their use reinforces the misconception that differences in social inequities or other factors are caused by innate biological differences and diverts attention from addressing the root causes of those social differences, which compromises the rigor and potential positive effect of the research.

Conclusion 4-3. Current practices in genetics studies often seem to reinforce typological views of human genetic ancestry (e.g., use of continental ancestry groups). Therefore, new models that reflect a more complex and realistic portrait of genetic ancestry are needed (e.g., genetic similarity).

Conclusion 4-4. The requirement to report participant demographics using OMB categories has perpetuated misconceptions or exacerbated typological thinking and can undermine the selection of variables that are most appropriate for a given genomics study.

Conclusion 4-5. Although perhaps useful for some analyses, the concept of genetically differentiated, discrete populations that are static in place and time does not apply to humans. For example, the racial and ethnic categories established by the OMB presume stable, fixed populations (even though the OMB categories themselves have changed over time), which makes them both inadequate and inaccurate for the purpose of representing human genetic variation.

Recommendation 1. Researchers should not use race as a proxy for human genetic variation. In particular, researchers should not assign genetic ancestry group labels to individuals or sets of individuals based on their race, whether self-identified or not.

Recommendation 2. When grouping people in studies of human genetic variation, researchers should avoid typological thinking, including the assumption and implication of hierarchy, homogeneity, distinct categories, or stability over time of the groups.

Recommendation 3. Researchers, as well as those who draw on their findings, should be attentive to the connotations and impacts of the terminology they use to label groups.

- As an example, the term *Caucasian* should not be used because it was originally coined to convey white supremacy,[1] and is often mistakenly interpreted today as a "scientific" term, thus erroneously conferring empirical legitimacy to the notion of a biological white race.
- Another example of a term that should not be used is *black race* because it wrongly implies the existence of a discrete group of human beings, or race, who could be objectively identified as "black."

These recommendations invoke the guiding principles of *respect, beneficence, equity and justice*, and *validity and reproducibility*. To promote validity through the use of accurate descriptors, the committee does not advocate the use of typological categories, such as the racial and ethnic categories established by the OMB in its Statistical Directive 15, for most purposes in human genomics research (see Chapter 5 for more specific guidance on the use of population descriptors). While the committee recognizes that the use of these categories, such as *white* or *Hispanic*, may be required of researchers under certain circumstances (for example, in describing participants in studies receiving U.S. federal funding), the fundamentally sociopolitical origins of these categories make them a poor fit for capturing human biological diversity (OMB, 1997). Even so, the required uses of OMB and other typological categories for certain reporting purposes need not dictate their use as analytical tools in human genomics research.[2] If nothing else, the OMB categories are impractical because they change over time in the wake of administrative decisions and cultural shifts.[3] Instead, the committee recommends that to evoke respect and beneficence, researchers who identify race as a valid population descriptor in a given study should reflect carefully on (1) the information that racial labels ostensibly provide, (2) whether such information—for example, on exposure to racial discrimination—might be better captured by other data (e.g., self-reports of such experiences), and (3) which labels or groupings would be most useful and

---

[1] Johann Friedrich Blumenbach (1752-1840) named Europeans "Caucasian" because he felt the most beautiful skull in his collection came from the Caucasus region and was thus a fitting symbol for a superior race (Marks, 1995; Painter, 2010).

[2] For a comprehensive study of such "categorical alignment"—e.g., "the merging of social categories from the worlds of medicine, social movements, and state administration"—see Epstein, Steven. *Inclusion: The Politics of Difference in Medical Research*, University of Chicago Press, 2007.

[3] For a longer history of changing U.S. Census racial categories, see Lee (1993) and Liebler et al. (2017).

informative for the study at hand. For example, the "black" racial label would not be useful in a study within the United States, because people who self-identify as "black" have a wide variety of national origins, class, and even linguistic backgrounds (Hamilton, 2019). In addition, this recommendation addresses problems inherent to the use of continental ancestry groupings. To adhere to equity and justice, alternative procedures that do not assume discrete continental ancestries are more valid and conceptually coherent; such alternatives are preferable and have the benefit of not reifying race. In Chapter 5, recommended use for specific population descriptors will be explored in greater detail.

ENVIRONMENTAL FACTORS

Nongenetic factors and contexts must be considered when examining genetic effects. Nongenetic factors—that is, anything that is not captured by inherited DNA variation—include environmental factors. Environmental factors are variable across individuals and include physical, chemical, and biological exposures; behavioral patterns; social context; and "life events," among others (Glass and McAtee, 2006; Ottman, 1996). Such environmental exposures can act on a phenotype on their own or do so by interplay with genetic effects (Seabrook and Avison, 2010) (see Chapter 2). These environmental effects, whether genome independent or dependent, may be themselves additive or multiplicative to a postulated genetic effect (Hunter, 2005). The critical importance of identifying environmental effects is that they improve or even alter researchers' understanding of the causal pathways to human genetic disease, thereby curtailing the common practice of assuming genetic causes for unexplained population differences in outcomes (Duello et al., 2021).

Environmental exposures are not always easy to identify or measure. As a shortcut, some epidemiologic and genetics studies have used race or ethnicity as a proxy for the environment without directly measuring specific factors (Benmarhnia et al., 2021; Duello et al., 2021; Evans et al., 2021). This is unfortunate since any two groups vary with respect to both the frequency of genetic variants and pertinent environmental exposures, and just as there are genetic differences between any two humans so are there individual-specific exposures and other environmental differences (Boardman et al., 2013; Johannesson et al., 2011).

In recent times, there have been efforts to understand the "exposome," representing the total suite of exposures and being the other major contributor to phenotypes besides the genome (Zhou and Lee, 2021). Additionally, the ability to quantify the epigenome, which can also be a measure of past environmental exposures, has improved (Cazaly et al., 2019). Considerable research is needed though to assess the usefulness of epigenetic markers as specific exposure sentinels. The 2011 National Academies report on precision medicine incorporated the exposome in its integrative knowledge network that provided the foundation for the U.S. Precision Medicine Initiative (NRC, 2011). Exposome studies are still rare and underused in genetics.

Conclusions and Recommendation

Conclusion 4-6. Genetic variation alone is not sufficient to describe or understand human phenotypes; environmental variation should also be examined when feasible.

Conclusion 4-7. Race, ethnicity, and other descent-associated population descriptors are poor proxies for environmental variables in human genetics studies.

Conclusion 4-8. In the absence of measured environmental factors, researchers often wrongly attribute unexplained phenotypic variance between populations to unmeasured genetic differences.

Recommendation 4. Researchers conducting human genetics studies should directly evaluate the environmental factors or exposures that are of potential relevance to their studies, rather than rely on population descriptors as proxies. If it is not possible to make these direct measurements and it is necessary to use population descriptors as proxies, researchers should explicitly identify how the descriptors are employed and explain why they are used and are relevant. Genetics and genomics researchers should collaborate with experts in the social sciences, epidemiology, environmental sciences, or other relevant disciplines to aid in these studies, whenever possible.

These recommendations are supported by the guiding principles of *equity and justice, validity and reproducibility,* and *transparency and replicability.* To promote validity and reproducibility, genetics and genomics researchers should collaborate with experts in the social sciences, epidemiology, environmental sciences, or other relevant disciplines if they are unsure about whether or how to include environmental variables in their studies. Transparency and replicability are key if descent-associated population descriptors are deemed necessary as proxies for the environment. In these cases, investigators must be transparent about how the descriptors are being used and why environmental factors were not able to be measured by other means. Equity and justice are evoked when researchers are clear about how and why a descent-associated population descriptor is being used as a proxy for environment. Such clarification will reduce the likelihood that the descriptor, rather than environment, will be viewed as the causal factor in any identified variance.

If investigators are unable to collaborate with experts who measure environmental effects, they can use existing resources to facilitate incorporation of exposure assessment into their studies. Some examples of these resources include the Human Health Exposure Analysis Resource,[4] National Institute of Environmental Health Sciences (Cui et al., 2022), the Centers for Disease Control and Prevention and National Institute for Occupational Safety and Health's resources on exposome and exposomics,[5] PhenX Toolkit,[6] and the *All of Us* Research Program's survey questions.[7] In future studies that collect new data, investigators should collect rich information on environmental exposures and social contexts. Some examples of information to collect may include geospatial data, socioeconomic position, dietary practices, education, and frequency of medical care. Moreover, whenever possible, the spatial and temporal distributions of measured environmental variables should be accounted for in combination with individual characteristics.

COMMUNITY ENGAGEMENT

My primary care clinician refers to me as an African American woman, yet I've never had a discussion with her or been asked about my ethnicity. So when I think about the absence of this discussion, I also begin to feel unseen and question what has been missed in the exchanges that I have with my provider because of the lack of having this conversation.
—Julia Ortega, testimony to the committee
in a public session on April 4, 2022

In a sense, it doesn't really matter what you call it, it matters who is doing the naming and who is in charge of providing agency, who is in control of the data, and who is in governance of that data, and how does that work... So deferring to communities to self-identify their belongingness is...a great step forward.
—Keolu Fox, testimony to the committee
in a public session on April 4, 2022

When we think about what's really called for and why we cannot abandon this very important project, it's because we need not only the contribution

---

[4] https://hhearprogram.org/ (accessed January 3, 2023).
[5] https://www.cdc.gov/niosh/topics/exposome/default.html (accessed January 3, 2023).
[6] https://www.phenxtoolkit.org/ (accessed January 3, 2023).
[7] https://databrowser.researchallofus.org/ (accessed January 3, 2023).

of genetic data information from people to research, but from research back to people who can use it.

—Donna Cryer, testimony to the committee
in a public session on April 4, 2022

In this report, a community is considered a group of people who have a common characteristic or are living in the same place. The committee acknowledges that how a community defines itself is dynamic. How researchers and community members define the community has implications for who is included in community engagement efforts. Community engagement can be a challenging and labor-intensive process, requiring resources including time, dedicated funding, and people with the necessary knowledge and skills (CTSA Consortium, 2011). It should be noted that the increased demands of community-engaged research also fall on research participants, potentially increasing the burden on their time.

Community engagement goals will vary depending on the research question, the participating community, and the researchers. Community engagement processes are diverse, and partners can include various organized groups such as agencies, institutions, or individuals (CTSA Consortium, 2011). The process may also be seen as a continuum of community involvement, stemming from study conception to translation and communication of findings, and the specific practices may also vary at different stages of the study, such as during research approval or guidance, sharing information, or consent (CTSA Consortium, 2011). Communities not only vary in how individuals and groups self-identify but also in their preferences for involvement (CTSA Consortium, 2011). Collaboration with individuals or groups begins by working with relevant parties from the community to identify their preferences on how, when, and to what extent they would like to be involved (CTSA Consortium, 2011). From there, researchers and community members can develop an engagement plan for the duration of the research, drawing on existing models and best practices to support community-engaged research (Beaton et al., 2017; Lemke et al., 2022; Minkler and Wallerstein, 2011; Wallerstein and Duran, 2010). Other resources include the National Institutes of Health (NIH) and Centers for Disease Control and Prevention Principles of Community Engagement[8] (NIH, 2015), the NIH Tribal Health Research Office,[9] and the Patient-Centered Outcomes Research Institute's engagement assessment tools[10] for ways to evaluate engagement at key stages of research (Sheridan et al., 2017). When community engagement is difficult or impossible (as with legacy samples),

---

[8] https://www.atsdr.cdc.gov/communityengagement/pdf/PCE_Report_508_FINAL.pdf (accessed January 3, 2023).

[9] https://dpcpsi.nih.gov/thro (accessed January 3, 2023).

[10] See https://www.pcori.org/engagement/engagement-resources/Engagement-Tool-Resource-Repository/engagement-assessment-tool (accessed January 3, 2023).

then proxy groups, who could be potential interested parties, could be used. Before legacy samples are used or relabeled, it is the researcher's responsibility to ensure that the samples were collected ethically and that the current related or proxy community groups agree to the use of these descriptors within the research design.

Frequently, descent-associated population descriptors (such as race) are assigned to samples by a researcher or clinician, leaving individuals and communities out of the conversations about what labels are applied to or preferred for their data (Lemke et al., 2022). Community engagement can improve communication, study coordination, and long-term collaborations between researchers and communities for enhancing that research (CTSA Consortium, 2011). Falling short of engaging and understanding communities and the relevant parties can undermine trust and the trustworthiness of research and, importantly, hamper delivery of the research outcomes to the communities whom researchers are trying to serve (Lemke et al., 2022). Effectively engaging communities requires multidisciplinary approaches that draw on expertise in history, sociology, anthropology, communication, and other fields working alongside the study's primary investigators in genetics and genomics (CTSA Consortium, 2011).

Conclusions and Recommendation

Conclusion 4-9. Community engagement recognizes the expertise of communities and relies on collaboration between researchers and the communities they are trying to serve.

Conclusion 4-10. Engaging participants in genomics research design increases the likelihood that population labels will respectfully describe participants, reduce potential harms, and lead to more beneficial science and translation to health and health care.

Conclusion 4-11. Lack of transparency by researchers threatens the trustworthiness of the entire research enterprise and may undermine goals of equity and justice by disenfranchising minoritized groups from participating.

Conclusion 4-12. Communities are dynamic and changing entities; therefore, with each new study, it is important to consider how the community being asked to participate in research could share in the selection of population descriptors.

Recommendation 5. Researchers, especially those who collect new data or propose new courses of study for a data set, should work in ongo-

ing partnerships with study participants and community experts to integrate the perspectives of the relevant communities and to inform the selection and use of population descriptors.

This recommendation supports the guiding principles of *respect, beneficence, equity and justice, validity and reproducibility,* and *transparency and replicability.* Equity and justice are invoked by engaging communities in the research process to avoid reproducing hierarchical thinking and to consider biases that may produce inequities. Through partnerships with participants and communities, researchers will gain a better understanding of their perspectives, needs, and expectations, which can foster or enhance a commitment to beneficence, not only pertaining to the research, but also in other meaningful ways. Validity and reproducibility are instituted by including the expertise of communities in determining the valid use of population descriptors and the risks and benefits associated with the research. Researchers should also partner with experts on engagement approaches to ensure community engagement occurs in a culturally sensitive way. Integrating team members who have knowledge and understanding of community perspectives early in study conception and throughout the research process is critical for achieving the goals of trustworthy science.

Respect is demonstrated through the inclusion of the community in the decision-making and study design processes when either collecting new data or using legacy data and by seeking information directly from the community. Although consulting communities about population descriptors is easier in studies collecting new data, it is important to also engage communities when using legacy data. This engagement might look different since the participants cannot be identified; however, proxy groups can be formed to discuss appropriate and preferred terms and usage of descriptors. Using the population descriptor preferences of individual and community participants reflects the principle of respect. However, if deviations from these preferred descriptors occur, respect and transparency must go hand in hand. In this case, transparency and replicability with communities mean communicating and explaining why the selected population descriptors differ from the participants' preferences, which helps preserve research relationships and allows individuals to make an informed decision about continued participation. Best practices for communicating technical and cultural concepts should be incorporated to increase transparent collaboration. Transparency and clear communication regarding the choices, rationale, and implications about decisions on descent-associated population descriptors promote trust and trustworthiness of the research and researchers. Individuals and communities called upon to participate in research must feel confident that researchers are committed to communicating their process.

REFERENCES

Beaton, A., M. Hudson, M. Milne, R. V. Port, K. Russell, B. Smith, V. Toki, L. Uerata, P. Wilcox, K. Bartholomew, and K. Bartholomew. 2017. Engaging Māori in biobanking and genomic research: A model for biobanks to guide culturally informed governance, operational, and community engagement activities. *Genetics in Medicine* 19(3):345-351.

Benmarhnia, T., A. Hajat, and J. S. Kaufman. 2021. Inferential challenges when assessing racial/ethnic health disparities in environmental research. *Environmental Health* 20(1):7.

Boardman, J. D., J. Daw, and J. Freese. 2013. Defining the environment in gene-environment research: Lessons from social epidemiology. *American Journal of Public Health* 103(Suppl 1):S64-S72.

Byeon, Y. J. J., R. Islamaj, L. Yeganova, W. J. Wilbur, Z. Lu, L. C. Brody, and V. L. Bonham. 2021. Evolving use of ancestry, ethnicity, and race in genetics research—a survey spanning seven decades. *American Journal of Human Genetics* 108(12):2215-2223.

Cazaly, E., J. Saad, W. Wang, C. Heckman, M. Ollikainen, and J. Tang. 2019. Making sense of the epigenome using data integration approaches. *Frontiers in Pharmacology* 10.

CTSA (Clinical Translational Science Awards) Consortium, and Community Engagement Key Function Committee Task Force on the Principles of Community Engagement. 2011. *Principles of community engagement (2nd edition).* Department of Health and Human Services.

Cui, Y., K. M. Eccles, R. K. Kwok, B. R. Joubert, K. P. Messier, and D. M. Balshaw. 2022. Integrating multiscale geospatial environmental data into large population health studies: Challenges and opportunities. *Toxics* 10(7):403.

Duello, T. M., S. Rivedal, C. Wickland, and A. Weller. 2021. Race and genetics versus 'race' in genetics: A systematic review of the use of African ancestry in genetic studies. *Evolution, Medicine, and Public Health* 9(1):232-245.

Evans, L., M. Engelman, A. Mikulas, and K. Malecki. 2021. How are social determinants of health integrated into epigenetic research? A systematic review. *Social Science in Medicine* 273:113738.

Fang, H., Q. Hui, J. Lynch, J. Honerlaw, T. L. Assimes, J. Huang, M. Vujkovic, S. M. Damrauer, S. Pyarajan, J. M. Gaziano, S. L. DuVall, C. J. O'Donnell, K. Cho, K.-M. Chang, P. W. F. Wilson, P. S. Tsao, J. M. Gaziano, R. Ramoni, J. Breeling, K.-M. Chang, G. Huang, S. Muralidhar, C. J. O'Donnell, P. S. Tsao, S. Muralidhar, J. Moser, S. B. Whitbourne, J. V. Brewer, J. Concato, S. Warren, D. P. Argyres, B. Stephens, M. T. Brophy, D. E. Humphries, N. Do, S. Shayan, X.-M. T. Nguyen, S. Pyarajan, K. Cho, E. Hauser, Y. Sun, H. Zhao, P. Wilson, R. McArdle, L. Dellitalia, J. Harley, J. Whittle, J. Beckham, J. Wells, S. Gutierrez, G. Gibson, L. Kaminsky, G. Villareal, S. Kinlay, J. Xu, M. Hamner, K. S. Haddock, S. Bhushan, P. Iruvanti, M. Godschalk, Z. Ballas, M. Buford, S. Mastorides, J. Klein, N. Ratcliffe, H. Florez, A. Swann, M. Murdoch, P. Sriram, S. S. Yeh, R. Washburn, D. Jhala, S. Aguayo, D. Cohen, S. Sharma, J. Callaghan, K. A. Oursler, M. Whooley, S. Ahuja, A. Gutierrez, R. Schifman, J. Greco, M. Rauchman, R. Servatius, M. Oehlert, A. Wallbom, R. Fernando, T. Morgan, T. Stapley, S. Sherman, G. Anderson, E. Sonel, E. Boyko, L. Meyer, S. Gupta, J. Fayad, A. Hung, J. Lichy, R. Hurley, B. Robey, R. Striker, Y. V. Sun, and H. Tang. 2019. Harmonizing genetic ancestry and self-identified race/ethnicity in genome-wide association studies. *American Journal of Human Genetics* 105(4):763-772.

Glass, T. A., and M. J. McAtee. 2006. Behavioral science at the crossroads in public health: Extending horizons, envisioning the future. *Social Science & Medicine* 62(7):1650-1671.

Green, E. D., C. Gunter, L. G. Biesecker, V. Di Francesco, C. L. Easter, E. A. Feingold, A. L. Felsenfeld, D. J. Kaufman, E. A. Ostrander, W. J. Pavan, A. M. Phillippy, A. L. Wise, J. G. Dayal, B. J. Kish, A. Mandich, C. R. Wellington, K. A. Wetterstrand, S. A. Bates, D. Leja, S. Vasquez, W. A. Gahl, B. J. Graham, D. L. Kastner, P. Liu, L. L. Rodriguez, B. D. Solomon, V. L. Bonham, L. C. Brody, C. M. Hutter, and T. A. Manolio. 2020. Strategic vision for improving human health at the forefront of genomics. *Nature* 586:683-692.

Hamilton, T. G. 2019. *Immigration and the remaking of black America*. Russell Sage Foundation.
Harawa, N. T., and C. L. Ford. 2009. The foundation of modern racial categories and implications for research on black/white disparities in health. *Ethnicity & Disease* 19(2):209.
Hunter, D. J. 2005. Gene–environment interactions in human diseases. *Nature Reviews Genetics* 6(4):287-298.
Johannesson, S., S. M. Rappaport, and G. Sallsten. 2011. Variability of environmental exposure to fine particles, black smoke, and trace elements among a Swedish population. *Journal of Exposure Science & Environmental Epidemiology* 21(5):506-514.
Jorde, L. B., and S. P. Wooding. 2004. Genetic variation, classification and 'race'. *Nature Genetics* 36(11 Suppl):S28-S33.
Lee, S. M. 1993. Racial classifications in the US Census: 1890–1990. *Ethnic and Racial Studies* 16(1):75-94.
Lee, S. S. J., J. Mountain, B. Koenig, R. Altman, M. Brown, A. Camarillo, L. Cavalli-Sforza, M. Cho, J. Eberhardt, M. Feldman, R. Ford, H. Greely, R. King, H. Markus, D. Satz, M. Snipp, C. Steele, and P. Underhill. 2008. The ethics of characterizing difference: Guiding principles on using racial categories in human genetics. *Genome Biology* 9(7).
Lemke, A. A., E. D. Esplin, A. J. Goldenberg, C. Gonzaga-Jauregui, N. A. Hanchard, J. Harris-Wai, J. E. Ideozu, R. Isasi, A. P. Landstrom, A. E. R. Prince, E. Turbitt, M. Sabatello, S. A. Schrier Vergano, M. R. G. Taylor, J.-H. Yu, K. B. Brothers, and N. A. Garrison. 2022. Addressing underrepresentation in genomics research through community engagement. *American Journal of Human Genetics* 109(9):1563-1571.
Lewontin, R. C. 1972. The apportionment of human diversity. In *Evolutionary biology*. Vol. 6, edited by T. Dobzhansky, M. K. Hecht, and W. C. Steere. New York: Springer. Pp. 381-398.
Liebler, C. A., S. R. Porter, L. E. Fernandez, J. M. Noon, and S. R. Ennis. 2017. America's churning races: Race and ethnicity response changes between census 2000 and the 2010 census. *Demography* 54(1):259-284.
Manica, A., F. Prugnolle, and F. Balloux. 2005. Geography is a better determinant of human genetic differentiation than ethnicity. *Human Genetics* 118:366-371.
Marks, J. 1995. *Human biodiversity: Genes, race, and history*. New York: Aldine de Gruyter.
Minkler, M., and N. Wallerstein. 2011. *Community-based participatory research for health: From process to outcomes*. 2nd ed. San Francisco, CA: John Wiley & Sons.
NIH (National Institutes of Health). 2015. *Principles of community engagement, second edition*. www.atsdr.cdc.gov/communityengagement/pdf/PCE_Report_508_FINAL.pdf (accessed January 17, 2023).
NRC (National Research Council). 2011. *Toward precision medicine: Building a knowledge network for biomedical research and a new taxonomy of disease*. Washington, DC: National Academies Press.
OMB (U.S. Office of Management and Budget). 1997. *Revisions to the standards for the classification of federal data on race and ethnicity*. https://www.whitehouse.gov/wp-content/uploads/2017/11/Revisions-to-the-Standards-for-the-Classification-of-Federal-Data-on-Race-and-Ethnicity-October30-1997.pdf (accessed December 6, 2022).
Ottman, R. 1996. Gene–environment interaction: Definitions and study designs. *Preventive Medicine* 25(6):764-770.
Painter, N. I. 2010. *The history of white people*. New York: W. W. Norton.
Popejoy, A. B. 2021. Too many scientists still say caucasian. *Nature* 596:463.
Romualdi, C., D. Balding, I. S. Nasidze, G. Risch, M. Robichaux, S. T. Sherry, M. Stoneking, M. A. Batzer, and G. Barbujani. 2002. Patterns of human diversity, within and among continents, inferred from biallelic DNA polymorphisms. *Genome Research* 12(4):602-612.
Seabrook, J. A., and W. R. Avison. 2010. Genotype–environment interaction and sociology: Contributions and complexities. *Social Science & Medicine* 70(9):1277-1284.

Sheridan, S., S. Schrandt, L. Forsythe, T. S. Hilliard, and K. A. Paez. 2017. The PCORI engagement rubric: Promising practices for partnering in research. *Annals of Family Medicine* 15(2):165-170.

Shim, J. K., S. L. Ackerman, K. W. Darling, R. A. Hiatt, and S. S. J. Lee. 2014. Race and ancestry in the age of inclusion: Technique and meaning in post-genomic science. *Journal of Health and Social Behavior* 55(4):504-518.

Wallerstein, N., and B. Duran. 2010. Community-based participatory research contributions to intervention research: The intersection of science and practice to improve health equity. *American Journal of Public Health* 100(Suppl 1):S40-S46.

Weiss, K. M., and B. W. Lambert. 2014. What type of person are you? Old-fashioned thinking even in modern science. *Cold Spring Harbor Perspectives in Biology* 6:a021238.

Zhou, X., and S. H. Lee. 2021. An integrative analysis of genomic and exposomic data for complex traits and phenotypic prediction. *Scientific Reports* 11:21495.

5

Guidance for Selection and Use of Population Descriptors in Genomics Research

INTRODUCTION

This chapter's primary audience are researchers who work with genetic data. The committee's intent is to provide practical guidance for using descent-associated population descriptors in human genetics and genomics research. As emphasized throughout the report, the appropriate population descriptor depends on the scientific question being asked. In some cases, none of these descriptors may be needed. In other situations, when descent-associated population descriptors are advisable or needed for methodological reasons, this chapter gives guidance on which approaches to consider and why.

In formulating these recommendations, the committee recognizes that there exists a large amount of legacy data in which study participants have already been classified on the basis of population descriptors (Khan et al., 2022; Wallace et al., 2020). When using such data, researchers may be constrained in their options, but their choices need to be described in ensuing publications. Furthermore, the committee appreciates the dynamic nature of research and the changing landscape of descent-associated population descriptors; there is no single solution to this challenge of appropriate use of descriptors, and applying a uniform approach across different types of studies is not possible. Rather, responsive approaches are needed to accommodate the specific research question being asked, develop best practices for grouping individuals and naming those groups, and take community preferences into account.

This chapter builds on the foundation established by the previous four chapters. Therefore, the committee encourages a careful reading of Chapters

1 through 4 in order to understand the context of these recommendations. Notably, Chapter 3 provides a set of guiding principles for conducting human genetics research (and all research involving humans) that support the report's recommendations and can help guide researchers when none of the specific best practices apply.

THE IMPORTANCE OF TRANSPARENCY AND SPECIFICITY WHEN SELECTING AND REPORTING POPULATION DESCRIPTORS

Transparency in methodology is a scientific norm for replication of research findings (NASEM, 2019), yet the challenge of transparency is not only in scientific description but also in communicating specifically how and why particular decisions were made. Although imperfect, categories and labels are needed to conduct and communicate science. Transparency, therefore, requires stating the rationale behind the classification scheme and group labels applied when using population descriptors. Beyond describing the exact nature of the study conducted and ensuring reproducibility, comparability and meta-analysis with other studies, transparency about methods, assumptions, and decision making promotes trustworthiness of the research (Claw et al., 2018; NASEM, 2019). Moreover, understanding the factors that inform decision making supports reproducibility.

When communicating their research methods, findings, and conclusions, researchers should be as transparent as possible about the specific procedures used to identify and name groups within their data sets. Transparency can take three major forms:

1. Clear identification of the concept of human difference underpinning the population descriptor(s) chosen for analysis, and the rationale for that choice,
2. Verbal descriptions of how samples were collected and labeled, as well as the rationale for the decisions made; and
3. Sharing analysis scripts and decision rules used to transform per-individual metadata (e.g., responses to surveys) to the labels used in an analysis.

The primary focus of this chapter is on the first two, namely the conceptual approaches and specific language that enable appropriate and accurate use of population descriptors in genomics research. Furthermore, the guidance that follows is intended to provide researchers with best practices and the rationale for decision making, in alignment with the guiding principles outlined in Chapter 3 and in an effort to support the goal of promoting trustworthy research.

In delimiting their study participants, researchers inevitably make choices about which classification schemes or descriptors to use, which scale of resolution to consider, which specific group labels to apply, how to treat individuals with missing data, and so forth. Researchers may also be constrained to using group categories and labels adopted by others in order to allow for data aggregation or harmonization (Doiron et al., 2013; Khan et al., 2022; Wallace et al., 2020). A further challenge arises when such categories have been applied inconsistently, with a mixture of some individuals in a study labeled based on race, others based on ethnicity, and yet others based on geography. For instance, some researchers merge genomic data sets from different sources and assign individuals to clusters on the basis of genetic similarity to each other or to reference panels. Then they assign labels to individuals based on a characteristic that is frequent in the cluster or by using the labels from the reference panels. The number and size of the clusters that are detected in any given study depend on the sample composition. Moreover, the group labeling assigned to these clusters is often highly heterogeneous, borrowing terms from distinct classification schemes, at vastly different scales of resolution, such as *African* (a continental geographical location)/*African American* (an ethnicity), *East Asian* (a geographic location), and *Finnish* (a nationality). In that regard, it is worth noting that even when the labels are carried over from previous data collection, choices have to be made about what ancillary information to use and which subsets of individuals to combine and split in the new analysis.

CONCLUSION AND RECOMMENDATIONS

Conclusion 5-1. In employing population descriptors and assigning group labels in genetics studies, researchers tend to rely on existing and commonly used population classifications, often with unclear justification for their choices.

Recommendation 6. Researchers should tailor their use of population descriptors to the type and purpose of the study, in alignment with the guiding principles, and explain how and why they used those descriptors. Where appropriate for the study objectives, researchers should consider using multiple descriptors for each study participant to improve clarity.

Recommendation 7. For each descriptor selected, labels should be applied consistently to all participants. For example, if ethnicity is the descriptor, all participants should be assigned an ethnicity label, rather than labeling some by race, others by geography, and yet others by ethnicity or nationality. If researchers choose to use multiple descriptors, each descriptor should be applied consistently across all individuals in that study.

Recommendation 8. Researchers should disclose the process by which they selected and assigned group labels and the rationale for any grouping of samples. Where new labels are developed for legacy samples, researchers should provide descriptions of new labels relative to old labels.

To equip researchers with the information to follow these recommendations, the committee developed the following decision-making tools and best practices. These tools will be particularly helpful to reviewers of genetics and genomics research proposals to try to ensure consistent usage of terms and appropriate study designs.

TOOLS FOR SELECTING AND USING POPULATION DESCRIPTORS IN GENETICS AND GENOMICS RESEARCH

The table below and decision tree in Appendix D suggest which descent-associated population descriptors are most appropriate as analytical tools for each of the seven genetics study types outlined in this report. Note that each descriptor represents a particular *concept of difference* across populations. In other words, the recommendations in the decision tree and table focus on the conceptual building blocks that researchers should use in study design, data analysis, and reporting their results. While the conceptual structure of research naturally has implications for the language that scientists adopt, the tree and table are not intended to be a linguistic straitjacket or a checklist of acceptable words. Instead, the objective of the committee's guidelines is to encourage genetics researchers to consider, define, and delineate very carefully the concepts of human difference with which they are working, and to choose wording that transparently reflects the analytical steps taken.

These considerations are particularly salient with respect to *genetic ancestry*, which is not directly observable and is instead inferred from measures of genetic similarity. Therefore, the committee recommends that researchers relying on such measures explicitly refer to genetic similarity when describing their results, rather than the shorthand of genetic ancestry. An exception is for human evolutionary genetics studies explicitly aiming to learn about genetic ancestries over time or space. The committee recommends that when researchers borrow labels from ethnic, racial, political, or geographic classification schemes, they be explicit about their choice of descriptor. For all these reasons, the columns in Table 5-1 distinguish the concept of genetic ancestry from other population descriptors like ethnicity or geography.

Key Terminology for the Selection Guide

Throughout the rest of this chapter, a nuanced understanding of key terms and concepts introduced earlier in this report is necessary (summarized in Box 5-1). In the table and decision tree below, *population descrip-*

BOX 5-1
Key Terminology for This Chapter

Population descriptor: a concept or classification scheme that categorizes people into groups (or "populations") according to a perceived characteristic or dimension of interest. A few examples include race, ethnicity, and geographic location, although this is a non-exhaustive list.

Group label: name given to a population that describes or classifies it according to the dimension along which it was identified. An example is *French* as the label for a group identified by its members' possession of French nationality, where *nationality* is the population descriptor.

Ancestral recombination graph: for a set of individuals, the graph depicting the genetic ancestry lines (or paths) that trace back to their common genetic ancestors at every position in the genome.

Ancestry: a person's origin or descent, lineage, "roots," or heritage, including kinship. Examples of ancestry group labels include clan names or patronyms, but geographic, ethnicity, or racial labels are often used to denote groups whose members are presumed to share common ancestry.

Genetic ancestry: the paths through an individual's family tree by which they have inherited DNA from specific ancestors. Genetic ancestry can be thought of in terms of lines extending upwards in a family tree from an individual through their genetic ancestors (see Figure 2-1). Shared genetic ancestry arises from having genetic ancestors in common (that is, overlapping lines of ancestry). For a set of individuals, a fundamental representation of genetic ancestry is a structure called an ancestral recombination graph. In practice, shared genetic ancestry is typically inferred by some measure(s) of genetic similarity.

Genetic ancestry group: a set of individuals who share more similar genetic ancestries. In practice a genetic ancestry group is constituted based on some measure(s) of genetic similarity; Once a set is designated as a genetic ancestry group, its members are often assigned a geographic, ethnic, or other nongenetic label that is common among its members.

Genetic similarity: quantitative measure of the genetic resemblance between individuals that reflects the extent of shared genetic ancestry.

See Appendix B for further comments, definitions, and citations.

tors refer to conceptual classification schemes used to group people based on specific characteristics. The appropriate application of these concepts in particular study contexts is the primary focus of the recommendations to follow. Group labels are names given to groupings of individuals.

Many of the best practices recommended by the committee rely on understanding the distinctions between genealogical ancestry, genetic ancestry, genetic ancestry *group*, and genetic similarity. For a full background of these concepts, see the subsection "Ancestry" in Chapter 2. Briefly, genealogical ancestors refer to the collection of ancestors for an individual as found in a family tree, such as parents, grandparents, and so on (Mathieson and Scally, 2020; Rohde et al., 2004). Genetic ancestry refers to the paths through an individual's family tree by which they have inherited DNA from specific ancestors (Mathieson and Scally, 2020); it is inferred from measures of genetic similarity rather than directly observed (Mathieson and Scally, 2020). Genetic ancestry *groups* are usually defined by demarcating sets of people based on various measures of genetic similarity. Then these groups are often given a label derived from nongenetic characteristics, such as ethnicity, geography, or race. This mapping of nongenetic descriptors introduces additional assumptions (see Chapters 2 and 4). Moreover, it may suggest homogeneity of genetic and environmental effects within social categories where none exists.

In a number of contexts, reliance on, and reference to, ancestry groupings may be unnecessary for the goals of the study. For example, when matching the background allele frequencies of cases to controls, there is a need to identify a set of individuals who are genetically similar, but not to rely on inferences about their genetic ancestry. Likewise, identifying individuals who are genetically similar to each other or to a reference panel is usually sufficient to delimit a subset of participants for genome-wide association studies (GWAS). Although the distinction between genetic ancestry and genetic similarity may be subtle, it is nonetheless important to enable moving beyond fundamental misconceptions about population descriptors, particularly race and typological thinking.

> *Conclusion 5-2. Assigning ancestry group labels based on such descriptors as geography, ethnicity, or race is often scientifically unnecessary and may contribute to typological thinking (Coop, 2022). In particular, genetic ancestry group is commonly conflated with continental geography, which in turn often stands in for—and thereby reifies—race (Lewis et al., 2022).*

Orientation to the Selection Guide

We must aspire to research scholarship and assessments and treatments based on actual and not assumed genetic variation, and the social, historical, structural context in which the bodies and lives of the people that we're interested exist. That means assessing the patterns of diversity that reflect the distribution of human genetic variation across the globe, not proxies thereof.

—Agustín Fuentes, testimony to the committee
in a public session on April 4, 2022

As shown in Table 5-1, best practices in the use of population descriptors vary by study type for any non-disease or disease trait. The committee considered seven major study types: (1) gene discovery for Mendelian traits; (2) prediction for Mendelian traits; (3) gene discovery for complex and polygenic traits; (4) prediction for complex and polygenic traits; (5) elucidation of molecular, cellular, or physiological mechanisms; (6) studies of health disparities with genomic data; and (7) studies of human evolutionary history. For descriptions and examples of each type, see the section "Classification of Genomics Study Types" in Chapter 1. Population descriptors refer to conceptual frameworks for describing descent-associated differences across groups of people. First, careful consideration should be given to whether descent-associated population descriptors are needed at all. If needed, and once researchers identify the appropriate population descriptor or descriptors for the context of their study, they should apply group labels consistent with each concept to all study participants. For a given study, more than one concept may be appropriate, and studies may benefit from using multiple descriptors. For example, a project may incorporate both geography and ethnicity simultaneously to distinguish, say, Kurds in Iraq from Kurds in Turkey.

In some contexts, descent-associated population descriptors are used not as indicators of shared genetic ancestry but as proxies for shared environmental exposures (see "The Importance of Environmental Factors in Genetics and Genomics Research" in Chapter 2). This practice should be avoided where possible in favor of measuring the environmental variable directly. Nevertheless, when direct measurements are not possible, Table 5-1 indicates which population descriptors might be most appropriate. While *race* (or *racialized group*) may capture some shared exposure to racism and therefore may be suitable for some health disparities studies, it is a poor proxy for other environmental exposures and carries the risk of contributing to typological thinking. Therefore, the committee recommends *race* not be used outside of a subset of health disparities studies. Even in that context, the combination of information from other classification schemes (e.g., ethnicity and geography) may be more accurate. Moreover, should descent-associated population descriptors be used as proxies for environments, that research-design decision should be explicitly noted and its rationale explained.

Finally, readers should bear in mind that the recommendations in Table 5-1 apply to the *analytical* use of population descriptors—that is, as variables or other tools in analysis. The committee recognizes, however, that researchers may wish—or be obligated—to use population descriptors for other research-related activities, notably for constructing and/or describing samples of individuals whose genetic material is to be analyzed. In the interests of equity, justice, or the diversification of human genetic data and knowledge about it, researchers may choose to use race and/or ethnicity in order to identify individuals to be included in their studies (Oni-Orisan et al., 2021), and Table 5-1 is not meant to govern such sampling decisions or procedures. Even outside the realm of analysis, however, the committee encourages scientists to carefully consider whether race and/or ethnicity are the most conceptually appropriate and useful descriptors for the information they wish to capture, or the best guides to seeking a heterogeneous sample.

Population Descriptor Selection Guide

Table 5-1 is a highly condensed summary of the best practices described in this chapter. It should not be inferred to indicate in absolute terms what to use and not use in every circumstance. To use Table 5-1 effectively, the reader is advised to review the subsection "Key Terminology for the Selection Guide" above and consult the text describing the best practices for each specific study type in conjunction with viewing the table. In addition, the reader should note that Table 5-1 provides only a broad overview and summary of the best practices; additional considerations for decision making are outlined in the decision tree (Figure D-1 in Appendix D) and in the body of this report.

The text that follows explains what is summarized in the table and illustrated in the decision tree in Appendix D. Although the text does not cover every possible variation of the genetics study types, the intent is for the discussion and examples to allow researchers to understand why certain population descriptors are recommended or discouraged depending on the type of study and the goals of the research.

TABLE 5-1 Recommended Approaches for the Use of Population Descriptors by Genomics Study Type

This table should be read and interpreted in conjunction with the report text. Consult the decision tree in Appendix D for more information and Chapter 5 text for best practices for each study type. See also the terminology box preceding the table and descriptions of each study type in Chapter 1 section "Classification of Genomics Study Types." For any given study, the use of multiple descriptors may be preferable.

LEGEND

✚	Preferred population descriptor(s)	▬	Should not be used
❓	In some cases; refer to Ch. 5 text and the decision tree in Appendix D	E	Descriptors could be used if appropriate proxies for environmental, not genetic, effects

GENOMICS STUDY TYPE	Race	Ethnicity/ Indigeneity	Geography	Genetic Ancestry	Genetic Similarity	Notes
1: Gene Discovery - Mendelian Traits	▬	❓	❓	❓	✚	Similarity suffices as a genetic measure; at fine-scale, other variables may be useful
2: Trait Prediction - Mendelian Traits	▬	E	E	❓	✚	No population descriptors may be necessary for analysis
3: Gene Discovery - Complex Traits	▬	E	E	❓	✚	Similarity suffices as a genetic measure
4: Trait Prediction - Complex Traits	▬	E	E	❓	✚	Similarity suffices as a genetic measure
5: Cellular and Physiological Mechanisms	▬	E	E	▬	❓	No population descriptors may be necessary for analysis
6: Health Disparities with Genomic Data	E	E	E	❓	✚	Not all health disparities studies rely on descent-associated population groupings, so none may be necessary for analysis
7: Human Evolutionary History	▬	❓	✚	✚	✚	Reconstructing genetic ancestry may be of central interest

Study Type 1: Gene Discovery for Mendelian Traits

Sequence variants that underlie Mendelian diseases fall into two categories: de novo mutations and inherited ones. When the goal is identifying de novo mutations, as through family studies (e.g., Simons et al., 2013; Turner et al., 2017), no population descent-associated descriptors are necessarily needed to identify variants. In some contexts, it may nonetheless be helpful to provide population descriptors (e.g., current geographic location) for the families that were studied in order to enable identification of additional cases or study the geographical spread of new mutations (e.g., Wexler, 2004).

Conclusion 5-3. Where the goal is to describe families in which de novo mutations have been identified, the relevant information is likely much more finely scaled than broad categories like those labeled by continental ancestry (or other large-scale genetic ancestry) or by ethnicity.

Best Practice 1: To enable identification of additional cases, rather than using genetic ancestry or ethnicity, researchers should use categories based on kinship (e.g., recent genealogical ancestors), identity-by-descent information, or fine-scaled geographical or genetic similarity data.

Studies aimed at identifying Mendelian disease variants use not only pedigrees, but also collections of unrelated affected persons (loosely called cohorts). A small number of variants found in these affected persons will be de novo, but most will be inherited and of unknown functional significance and pathogenicity. To annotate such variants, researchers commonly rely on a reference database comprised of data from individuals who are not diagnosed with the disease, in order to exclude those variants that are likely unrelated to the condition. In doing so, the goal is to exclude variants that are not rare (e.g., common variants) found in groups of individuals or populations with genetic backgrounds similar to one another. Alternatively, researchers may rely on a global reference panel to evaluate whether the variant of interest is at high frequency anywhere in the world, and if so, exclude it as a likely causal mutation.

Best Practice 2: Where researchers aim to match the genomes of focal individuals to people that are genetically similar, they should not rely on matching solely by racial (e.g., black), ethnic (e.g., Hispanic), geographic (e.g., West African), or national (e.g., Nigerian) categorizations, which are poor proxies for allele frequencies. Since in this context researchers are not interested in genetic ancestry per se, the committee further recommends that, when possible, they avoid ancestry category labels (e.g., "Admixed-American" in the 1000 Genomes), as such labeling brings in additional, unnecessary assumptions (see Chapters 2 and 4). The committee recommends instead that they rely on genetic similarity measures to delimit the reference set to which to compare focal individuals and to describe study participants (Coop, 2022).

Study Type 2: Prediction for Mendelian Traits

Examples of phenotypic prediction for Mendelian traits include prenatal or newborn screening (e.g., for Tay Sachs or phenylketonuria—PKU, respectively) or clinical testing for highly penetrant germline mutations that increase disease risk (e.g., Tan et al., 2017). Once the genetic basis for a disease has been elucidated, group labels may no longer be needed as a stand-in for allele frequencies. Instead, people can readily be genotyped for the variants themselves. Furthermore, making screening for specific alleles available only in people with particular descriptors (e.g., Tay Sachs only in children of Ashkenazi Jewish parents) will miss some disease-variant carriers (Dolitsky et al., 2020; Nazareth et al., 2015). In clinical scenarios, there may be exceptions where allele frequencies are necessary to estimate the genotype of missing parents. Here again, genetic similarity is more appropriate than reference to genetic ancestry.

For some traits considered Mendelian (e.g., Huntington's disease), prognosis, for instance regarding the age of onset, depends on modifier alleles in the genome (GeM-HD Consortium, 2015). Where the modifier alleles are unknown, which they usually are today, information about genetic similarity may be helpful in providing some information about allele frequencies at other loci in the genome. When the modifier alleles are known, however, sequencing the individual will provide much more accurate individual information than will population descriptors.

> **Best Practice 3:** Where the genetic basis of a trait is known, researchers should focus on characterizing the individual's alleles rather than use population descriptors as an unreliable proxy for the genomic background.

Phenotypic trait prediction of Mendelian disorders may also depend on environmental factors, such as air pollution or secondhand smoke exposure for children with cystic fibrosis (O'Neal and Knowles, 2018). In such cases, researchers may be tempted to include such population descriptors as race, ethnicity, or geography to capture shared exposures (Martinez et al., 2022). However, where the aim is explicitly to measure environmental effects, the committee recommends that descent-associated population descriptors not be used in place of individual-level data, as the use of such descriptors runs the risk of erroneously suggesting that the effects of interest are genetic.

Best Practice 4: Given that any descent-associated population descriptor will be a poor proxy for environmental effects (Benmarhnia et al., 2021; Martinez et al., 2022), researchers should aim to directly collect information about as many potentially relevant environmental factors as possible.

Best Practice 5: When including population descriptors for phenotype prediction of Mendelian traits, researchers should be explicit about whether the aim is to study genetic or environmental effects or both, and whether these can be disentangled given the study design.

Study Types 3 and 4: Gene Discovery and Prediction for Complex and Polygenic Traits

Complex traits, such as height or the risk of a disease such as type 2 diabetes, depend on the effects of not only many loci across the genome but also the environment (Falconer and Mackay, 1996). In the past two decades, the main method to map the genetic basis of such traits has been genome-wide association studies of unrelated individuals (Hirschhorn and Daly, 2005). Such efforts have been motivated by two distinct goals: to identify loci that affect a particular phenotype, and to predict trait values in currently asymptomatic individuals (Visscher et al., 2017). Association studies are conducted in sets of individuals that have some degree of genetic similarity in order to better control for effects of alleles in the genomic background as well as potential environmental effects that correlate with the genomic background. How much of a problem environmental confounding presents depends on the trait (e.g., Okbay et al., 2022).

Study Type 3: Gene Discovery for Complex and Polygenic Traits

For researchers who are mapping variants that influence complex trait values, common practice is to describe their study participants as members of genetic ancestry groups that are labeled with geographic, ethnic, or racial terms. Such labels for inferred ancestry groups are defined at very different levels of resolution depending on the data at hand, such as the *Southern European* versus the *white British* subsample of the UK Biobank. Moreover, to increase their sample sizes when they lack access to the original data, researchers often combine summary statistics provided by different studies (Lesko et al., 2018). In that case, current practice usually consists of grouping them under a general label, such as *European*, without spelling out the often-implicit assumptions about genetic and environmental effects in the combined samples or considering the genetic or environmental diversity within any such group (Coop, 2022). In this context, researchers are not interested in ancestry or race per se, and instead are aiming to identify study participants who are more genetically similar to one another, to better control for effects of the genomic background and correlated environmental effects.

Similar considerations arise when conducting mapping studies in recently admixed individuals (Shriner, 2013; Thornton and Bermejo, 2014). In this context, the mapping is conducted by considering local ancestry estimates, that is, inferences based on genetic similarity for different segments of the genome (Atkinson et al., 2021). Included in the statistical model also are sometimes genome-wide ancestry proportions, estimates that capture genomic background effects beyond the scale of local ancestry estimates, and, sometimes, ethnic or racial labels as a proxy for environmental exposures.

Best Practice 6: When mapping variants that contribute to complex traits, the goal is to conduct the study in a set of individuals that are genetically more similar, rather than to infer ancestry per se. Therefore, researchers should characterize their study participants in terms of their genetic similarity to one another or to a reference panel, with a specified similarity measure (Coop, 2022).

As an example, researchers would describe samples as "carrying genotypes most genetically similar by measure X to the GBR panel of the 1000 Genomes data set, as compared to individuals sampled elsewhere in the world" (GBR being the acronym for British in England and Scotland) (Coop, 2022) or by using coordinates in a low-dimensional representation of the data, like principal component analysis (PCA) or uniform manifold approximation and projection (UMAP) (e.g., "individuals projecting to the region [-0.1,-0.05] in PC1 and [0.3,0.5] in PC2 of a PCA generated from the 1000 Genomes data set"). For recently admixed individuals, this description would then naturally lend itself to statements such as, "Seventy-three percent of the genome is most genetically similar to genotypes of individuals in the GBR panel, and 27 percent of the genome is most similar to genotypes of individuals in the YRI panel" (YRI being the acronym for Yoruba in Ibadan, Nigeria). (Or alternatively, "73% of the genome is most similar to genomes from region 1 and 27% from region 2 in a 1000 Genomes PCA.") This approach avoids descriptions of recently admixed people as either African or European when they derive recent ancestry from diverse locations in both continents. Importantly, this descriptive change does not alter or compromise the underlying science. For comparability across studies, there is still work to be done to assess which similarity method to use and how these may change with the composition of the reference panel and different choices of genotype measures.

Study Type 4: Prediction for Complex and Polygenic Traits

GWAS results can be useful for trait prediction, even where the mechanism linking genotypic variation to phenotypic variation is not understood (Torkamani et al., 2018). In particular, the hope is to use polygenic scores (PGS) to identify individuals at high risk for specific diseases (e.g., Khera et al., 2018; Mavaddat et al., 2019). PGS are calculated by summing alleles carried by an individual, weighted by effect sizes of alleles that are estimated in association studies (often GWAS); PGS provide a predictor of a deviation from a mean value in a given study population (often adjusted for relevant covariates, such as sex and age) (Sirugo et al., 2019).

Polygenic scores (also called polygenic risk scores) are based on GWAS that pick up not only causal loci but also genetic variants correlated with causal variants, to an extent that depends on allelic association (called linkage disequilibrium or LD) patterns among sites (Choi et al., 2020). Since at present causal variants can rarely be pinpointed, the construction of a PGS requires weighting all these associations. In practice, therefore, phenotypic prediction of complex traits relies on LD patterns characterized in a set of individuals that are genetically similar, by some operational definition.

When the goal is to predict trait values—as distinct from identifying causal loci—it may not be as important to entirely control for environmental effects on the trait that are correlated with genetic differences. In some contexts, uncontrolled environmental stratification can actually enhance predictive power (Mostafavi et al., 2020). For related reasons, the practice of performing genetic prediction after stratifying by a population descriptor can increase predictive power because it implicitly captures both genetic similarity and shared environmental exposures. A danger, though, is that by including a contribution of nongenetic effects into what is widely understood to be a genomic predictor, this practice will end up over-emphasizing the role of genetics in trait etiology and reifying group differences.

Another important aspect of genomic trait prediction is generalizability beyond the GWAS study population. Generalizability is particularly important because, to date, the vast majority of GWAS have been conducted by sampling people in Europe or those who report recent European ancestry (Martin et al., 2019; Mills and Rahal, 2020). Given that LD patterns vary across the globe (Charles et al., 2014), as do the frequencies of causal loci, the prediction accuracy of PGS is expected to decrease with genetic divergence from the GWAS set, even if nothing else were to differ (Wang et al., 2020, 2022). That decrease is seen in practice: PGS have lower prediction accuracy with increasing genetic distance from the GWAS set of individuals (Martin et al., 2019; Privé et al., 2022; Scutari et al., 2016; Wang et al., 2020). Factors other than LD and shifts in causal allele frequencies may also decrease prediction power, such as differences in the degree of environmental variance or gene–environment interactions; in other words, genetic effects may differ across environmental settings (Giannakopoulou et al., 2021; Mills and Rahal, 2020; Mostafavi et al., 2020; Wang et al., 2022).

> **Best Practice 7:** When predicting complex traits, the goal is to study a set of individuals that vary in a trait but are relatively similar genetically, rather than to infer ancestry per se. Therefore (as with Best Practice 5 and 6), researchers should characterize their study participants in terms of their genetic similarity (to one another or with regards to a reference panel), with a specified similarity measure (Coop, 2022).

Considerations Common to Gene Discovery and Prediction for Complex and Polygenic Traits

The committee recognizes that after delimiting study participants based on genetic similarity to a reference panel, researchers may want to refer to the set of study participants with a label based on ethnicity (e.g., Yoruba), nationality (e.g., Nigerian), or geography (e.g., residing in Nigeria)—or a combination of various labels—either as shorthand in communicating the results, or to underscore a particular characteristic of the group that distinguishes their ethnicity, geography, or demographic history from that of the closest other individuals in the reference panel. In so doing, care should be taken to avoid applying broad labels (e.g., African ancestry) to panels represented by narrower sampling (e.g., YRI). This consideration underscores the need for more widely available, geographically and ethnically diverse reference panels. In every case, researchers should be transparent about their reasons for using such ancestry labels and for the choice of the particular label(s) in question. Importantly, in many cases, it may be unnecessary to refer to genetic ancestry at all, since terms such as *the study population*, alongside information about how and where individuals were sampled, may be sufficient and require fewer assumptions.

The committee further appreciates that when researchers use summary statistics from a previous GWAS and have no access to the individual-level genotype and phenotype data (e.g., when conducting a meta-analysis), it is not always feasible to assess genetic similarity to a reference panel. In this case, researchers should be explicit about the reasons for the nomenclature they have adopted or borrowed (e.g., if grouping many sets of individuals under a common label) and the procedure by which individuals have been retained or excluded from the sample; where possible, they should adopt labels based on the use of genetic similarity. In this regard, those sharing data should also attempt to provide indirect measures of genetic similarity (e.g., summary statistics for coordinate positions in a reference principal component analysis) that might enable genetic similarity to be assessed more precisely than is possible with group labels.

Where no reference panel is available, researchers often use a group label based on an attribute that is common to the study participants, such as a subset of people who self-identify as "white British" in the UK Biobank. Researchers should be explicit about their reasons for choosing the attribute used to delineate and describe the study participants.

> **Best Practice 8:** Researchers should describe samples in as many dimensions as possible, using population descriptors, individual-specific environmental data, and their ascertainment scheme (e.g., were participants recruited from a research hospital, in an urban or rural area, and so on).

> **Best Practice 9:** When descent-associated descriptors such as ethnicity or geography are used, researchers should be explicit about what types of effects they intend to capture—genetic, nongenetic, or both—and whether the effects can be teased apart reliably given the study design.

> **Best Practice 10:** Where the goal is to control for environmental effects that are correlated with genomic background effects, researchers should, if possible, replace or, at least, augment the use of population descriptors with more reliable and precise measures of individual environmental effects. Whenever labels remain, researchers should be explicit about their reasons for using them.

Cataloging the data collection in these ways will enable samples to be assessed for their genetic similarity to reference panels as well as for their similarity along nongenetic dimensions such as employment status or geographic location. A richer description of the data will also help to identify obstacles to generalizability beyond genetic similarity. A further benefit may be that forms of study ascertainment or enrollment bias could potentially be taken into account (e.g., Van Alten et al., 2022).

Finally, a major goal of all of these genetics and genomics studies, particularly GWAS, is to dissect the genetic and environmental architecture of these traits, and to identify the underlying mechanisms (pathophysiology). Further progress along this front will almost surely require the collection of new samples with new data, particularly longitudinal data, rather than simply retrofitting legacy studies.

Study Type 5: Elucidation of Molecular,
Cellular, or Physiological Mechanisms

Many studies that include human genetic data ultimately aim to understand the molecular, cellular, tissue, and physiological underpinnings of traits, sometimes triggered by gene discovery. One example might be studies aimed at understanding the genetic and neuronal mechanisms by which a DNA repeat expansion causes Huntington's disease (Jimenez-Sanchez et al., 2017). Another is the molecular mechanism underlying messenger RNA (mRNA) vaccines against SARS-CoV-2: their development relied on an understanding of antibody production and chemical modifications to mRNA that help evade the human innate immune response, much of which was learned in mice, human cells, and other model systems (Delorey et al., 2021; Sadarangani et al., 2021). In such cases, where underlying mechanisms are expected to be shared by all humans (and often by other species), there is no compelling reason to stratify study participants by descent-associated population descriptors at all.

As noted by Pavlicev and Wagner (2002), "A shared mechanistic basis of a trait does not mean that exactly the same loci will be detectable by association with variation in this trait." Conversely, the observation that variation in a trait differs in its allelic basis among humans does not imply that the underlying mechanisms are different. Thus, despite the universality of the underlying mechanisms of vaccination (Delorey et al., 2021; Sadarangani et al., 2021), humans vary in their specific response (Randolph et al., 2021), likely because of both genetic variants and environmental exposures. As an example, in all humans, myopia is caused by deformations in the shapes of the eye or cornea and can be corrected by eyeglasses (Chakraborty et al., 2020). Nonetheless, the genetic and environmental factors that lead to myopia likely differ across the world, owing to changes in allele frequencies, average effect sizes, and environmental exposures (Chakraborty et al., 2020; Li and Zhang, 2017). Researchers may be interested in understanding such perturbations to the underlying mechanisms and how they are distributed geographically, but often the primary goal is to leverage these perturbations (e.g., loss-of-function mutations) as a tool to better understand underlying mechanisms.

When specific candidate loci or salient environmental factors are unknown, a common approach has been to use population descriptors, and in particular ancestry group labels, as a proxy for differences in allele frequencies across the genome and potentially environmental exposures. A danger of this approach is the implication, implicit or explicit, that the underlying mechanisms themselves somehow differ by population descriptors, when in fact, the observed differences are caused by alleles at specific loci in the genome or varying environmental exposures (or interactions of the two). Once the nature of the perturbations has been identified, any observed differences between groups defined by population descriptors will resolve as differences between individuals carrying distinct alleles and the environments to which they are exposed.

> *Conclusion 5-4. Given that underlying cellular and physiological mechanisms are expected to be universal among humans, the default practice in such studies should be to not use any descent-associated population descriptors.*

Best Practice 11: When researchers are interested in studying perturbations to underlying mechanisms that arise from genetic variation, and the genetic variants are *known*, population descriptors should not be used as a substitute for individual information. If, instead, the genetic variants are *unknown*, and researchers are interested in delimiting a set of individuals with similar allele frequencies, they should rely on genetic similarity rather than such descriptors as ethnicity or geography.

Best Practice 12: Where the goal is to study the effect of unknown environmental exposures or possible gene–environment interactions, researchers should aim to replace or supplement population descriptors with direct information about potentially salient environmental factors. Regardless, researchers should be explicit about their intent in using population descriptors, including whether the aim is to study genetic or environmental effects or both, and whether these can be teased apart given the study design.

Study Type 6: Studies of Health Disparities with Genomic Data

Health disparities studies often compare groups of individuals identified by different descent-associated population descriptors (e.g., by OMB racial and ethnic categories). Some of these studies include genetic information, such as genome-wide genotyping data (Batai et al., 2021), data for variants at a single locus (e.g., apolipoprotein E gene—APOE4) (Torres and Kittles, 2007), or tumor genome sequencing (Daly and Olopade, 2015; Spratt et al., 2016). Other health disparities studies include only nongenetic data but may assign the unexplained variance to untested genetic differences (e.g., Kistka et al., 2007).

> *Conclusion 5-5. It is invalid to assign unexplained trait variance to any type of effect without direct evidence; notably, racial or ethnic phenotypic differences cannot be ascribed to genetic differences without evidence. The unexplained variance could be caused by environmental factors that are not considered or were imprecisely or inaccurately measured, or by inadequacy of the statistical model used.*

Given the variety of goals and sources of input data for different health disparity studies, it is helpful to consider some of these categories separately. Below is a short but incomplete list of three types of health disparities study that include genetic and genomic data.

- <u>Health Disparities Study Type 1</u>: The sole goal is to study the role of one or multiple genetic variants on observed or possible health disparities between groups.

  Best Practice 13: In this type of study, what is needed is to consider the effects of the focal variant of interest among individuals with similar allele frequencies, so genetic similarity is the relevant descriptor to use, and racial and ethnic labels should not be used. The use of genetic similarity to a reference panel is both more accurate and more transparent than using descent-associated descriptors such as race or ethnicity (Coop, 2022).

  In cases where ancestries are correlated with traits such as skin color (Parra et al., 2004), which may mediate the effect of racism on health (Kittles et al., 2007; Teteh et al., 2020), genetic ancestry may be considered if these traits are a key component of the research question.

- <u>Health Disparities Study Type 2:</u> The goal is to study the effect of environmental exposures or examine possible gene–environment interplay.

  Best Practice 14: Researchers should avoid racial or ethnic labels because they are poor proxies for differences in environmental exposures. Instead, the committee recommends that they replace or supplement descent-associated population descriptors with information about the relevant factors that mediate differences in environmental exposures, such as education, types of employment, housing quality, and access to health care, to name only a few.

  There is one exception to Best Practice 14. When the goal is explicitly to study the effect of structural racism and discrimination, then racial and ethnic labels may be appropriate but need to be carefully described (e.g., self-identified or not) and justified. Instruments and variables that measure discrimination (e.g., Williams's Everyday

Discrimination Scale[1]) or mediators of discrimination directly may be more appropriate, although challenging to implement (Hardeman et al., 2022).

- Health Disparities Study Type 3: Although the goal is to study the effect of environmental exposures or examine possible gene–environment interplay, information about environmental factors is limited.

Best Practice 15: If environmental information is unavailable and population descriptors such as race or ethnicity are used as proxies for it in such studies, for example in analyses of electronic health records, then their source should be described in detail (e.g., self-reported or assigned by provider) and along multiple dimensions (e.g., Hispanic, Mexican-American, rural, sampled in Texas health clinic, born in Texas). Moreover, the researcher should explicitly state why each descent-associated population descriptor is being used, by identifying specifically what types of effects their inclusion is intended to capture and the accuracy of this capture.

Study Type 7: Studies of Human Evolutionary History

Population genetics studies of human history and prehistory aim to use genetics to make inferences about the genetic evolution of humans and integrate such inferences with data from archeology, history, paleontology, and other disciplines (e.g., Nielsen et al., 2017). Many such studies analyze variation data using models and methods that employ the mathematical construct of discrete, unstructured populations (Gutenkunst et al., 2009; Patterson et al., 2012; Pritchard et al., 2000). It is common practice also to rely on samples collected by geographic or ethnic criteria (e.g., Scheinfeldt et al., 2019).

Some studies of human evolutionary history embed all samples within the same analytic structure, notably when inferring an ancestral recombination graph (e.g., Schaefer et al., 2021). In that case, descent-associated population descriptors may not be necessary, such as when the goal is to estimate the time to the most recent common genetic ancestor of modern humans at a locus (Mallick et al., 2016).

Nonetheless, population descriptors will often be needed to describe the sample collection scheme to other researchers and to capture characteristics of sampled individuals that help place them in a historical and geographic context. These descriptors might include the geographic provenance of the

---

[1] See https://scholar.harvard.edu/davidrwilliams/node/32397 (accessed January 20, 2023).

sample, or some indicator of the geographic or ethnic affiliation of an individual's recent ancestors (e.g., via grandparental birthplace questionnaires, or by reference to ethnicity, such as "Houston residents who identify ethnically as Gujarati"). In many circumstances, a sample will be labeled by the ethnicity, current geographic location, or commonly spoken language of present-day people to which its genome bears the greatest genetic similarity (e.g., Yoruba, Andamanese, Basque).

Conclusion 5-6. In genetics studies of human evolutionary history, social or geographic population descriptors are often used to describe genetic ancestry groups inferred based on genetic similarity (e.g., labels may be based on shared characteristics of participants such as language spoken, self-identified ethnicity, or location sampled) in order to shed light on population history.

In studying human evolution, researchers may also be interested in studying the genetic and phenotypic changes that occurred in response to localized selection pressures. To study such biological adaptations, which occur through systematic changes in allele frequencies over generations in groups of individuals, researchers will often delimit a set of people whose ancestry is thought to have been subject to similar selection pressures at some time point (e.g., to study the evolution of lactose tolerance in descendants of Nilotic-speaking pastoralists from East Africa in the past several thousand years). A challenge is that the appropriate scale will often be unknown a priori. For example, in studying human adaptation to *Plasmodium vivax*, continental groupings likely do not offer the necessary fine-scale resolution. Then one must address whether to try to enrich specifically for individuals whose recent genetic ancestors lived in environments where *P. vivax* was common, or focus on individuals currently living in such environments, despite the fact that their ancestors may not have been subject to the same pressures.

Best Practice 16: When gathering new data in genetics studies of human evolutionary history, after researchers engage local communities as described in Chapter 4, they should collect and include population descriptors along multiple dimensions, both to convey the myriad ways in which an individual could be described and to enable additional uses of these samples in the future. Notably, in addition to genetic data, researchers should also report their sampling location and when known, their birthplace, parental birthplaces, language(s) spoken, and self-described ethnicity. However, researchers should be consistent with population descriptors used for all samples in a study (for example, it is not good practice to use self-identified ethnic group for some samples but geographic origin for others).

The committee appreciates that many researchers will use existing data and therefore inherit population descriptors that may not be of their design. In that case, researchers should be transparent about the specific criteria according to which they included or excluded individuals. Moreover, when using legacy data, researchers should be mindful to apply consistent population descriptors across samples within the study. New labels may be appropriate to define, and when doing so, the new labels and their relationship to previous ones should be communicated.

While not a focus of this report, the committee notes additional challenges can arise in assigning population descriptors in studies of ancient DNA, which often integrate genetic data with archeological, or even historical data, to make inferences about modern population origins. Individuals in such studies are often given population labels based on cultural practices inferred from material objects identified from archeological data (e.g., the Corded Ware and Yamnaya cultures) (Eisenmann et al., 2018). Assigning cultural population names to ancient individuals clustered together using genetic data can be problematic. As Eisenmann and colleagues note:

> Giving groups that have been identified through a completely different line of evidence—in this case material culture and genomics—the same or related names results in their conflation and the archaeological designations risk becoming reified in genetic terms (and vice versa) (Eisenmann et al., 2018).

Their recommendation is to either label genetically defined populations numerically (giving no cultural label) or use a mixed system where names are based on a combination of geographic and subsistence terms, and a relative time span, together with archeological culture when appropriate (Eisenmann et al., 2018). One example of such a label would be to describe individuals from present-day Spain and dating to the Early Neolithic period as "Spain_EN" (Eisenmann et al., 2018). Such practices are in general alignment with the principles outlined in this report, though the committee reiterates that consideration of the questions of interest when choosing what labels to use, if any, is paramount.

Decision Tree for the Use of Population Descriptors

To aid a researcher contemplating a specific genetics or genomics study, the committee believes that a decision tree to systematically decide which descent-associated population descriptors to consider using and which to avoid is a helpful addition to the table. The decision tree can be found in Appendix D. The process begins by asking the following questions:

1. What is the purpose of your study?
2. Are you collecting new data, working with existing individual-level data, or using summary-level legacy data?
3. Does your research question pertain to environmental sources of differences?
4. If the answer to question 3 is yes, then do you plan to study environmental effects as a predictor or as a control variable?

CONSIDERATIONS FOR HARMONIZATION OF POPULATION DESCRIPTORS ACROSS STUDIES

In general, harmonization enhances comparability of data among different studies and enables the continued use of existing data to answer new research questions (Doiron et al., 2013; Khan et al., 2022; Wallace et al., 2020). Harmonization of population descriptors, specifically, would allow greater interoperability among data sets in human genomics research. Although the advantages of harmonization are clear, there are many challenges to the harmonization of population descriptors (see "Challenges of Harmonization and Legacy Data" in Chapter 1). Descriptors differ not only in scale or resolution but also in the concepts they represent. For example, is it possible to harmonize studies where one uses race or ethnicity, another uses geography, and yet another genetic similarity? Another consideration is the harmonization of descriptors to account for both unique preferences and the needs analytical groups may have within the consortia (Lee et al., 2019). There is a fundamental tension between harmonization on one hand and flexibility or specificity on the other, and the solution is not straightforward. To cope with these challenges, informatics tools have been developed to harmonize data and metadata. Some examples include common data elements (see Box 5-2), machine learning algorithms, visualization tools, and data processing standards.

Over time, regularly employing the best practices and recommendations in this chapter will promote harmonization across studies. As illustrated through the best practices above, different descriptors may be warranted based on study design. Just as individual investigators should be mindful of the purpose of their study, harmonization efforts similarly need to consider research objectives since the context shapes the appropriate use of population descriptors. The objective is less to offer a single definitive descriptor or set of labels but rather systems and approaches for harmonization—that is, clear ways to denote which population descriptors are used and why and how to merge data sets that may have used different descriptor schemes.

BOX 5-2
Common Data Elements for Researchers to Include as
Metadata to Help Harmonize Across Studies

Systems for improving data sharing and harmonization are an important research need. When sharing data, researchers could explicitly share a set of accessory files that provide information to communicate their labeling schemes. An example of useful common data elements to include would be:

Per population descriptor:
- Overall rationale for the population descriptor (e.g., classification scheme) and associated group labels
- Set of possible population descriptor values (e.g., group labels) and recommended abbreviations of label values used in study
- Per individual in the study:
  - Label value
  - Provenance of label value: Self-report, ascribed externally and by whom, other
- When using existing data, if a new set of population descriptor values (e.g., group labels) is being used instead of those used in the original data set, provide a mapping of how old labels map onto new labels.

For example, for geographic population descriptors:
- Identification of specific geographic labeling scheme (e.g., based on sample location, birthplace)
- If relevant, set of geographic entities with associated shape files defining boundary of the entity or latitude/longitude specifying representative locations
- Per individual either:
  - Point based:
    - Latitude
    - Longitude
    - Estimated mean square error in units of kilometers
    - Provenance: Self-reported, ascribed externally, other
  - Geographic entity based:
    - Entity value
    - Provenance: Self-report, ascribed externally, other

Upholding the principle of transparency and adhering to Recommendations 6, 7, and 8 inherently support harmonization through the application of consistent definitions of population descriptors and transparent communication of methods. More specifically, for novel data collection, data should be collected per individual along multiple nongenetic dimensions and population descriptor types that may facilitate other studies. In addition, clear instructions should be provided on how downstream users can respect consent and any collaborative agreements with study participants regarding population descriptors. For existing individual-level data, the available metadata can be used while following existing agreements and consent structures to form the population descriptors (see the decision tree in Appendix D).

Harmonized population descriptors that are well understood would be highly valuable. In the context of genetics studies, genetic similarity to specific reference sets could have advantages for promoting harmonization. While a broader sampling of human genetic diversity is needed, current candidates for specific reference sets include, for example, data from the 1000 Genomes Project, the Human Genome Diversity Project, and the Simons Genome Diversity Project (1000 Genomes Project Consortium et al., 2015; Bergström et al., 2020; Cann et al., 2002; Mallick et al., 2016).

A specific challenge is harmonizing across studies so readers of a research manuscript can understand a label quickly and in a technically precise way. For example, a possible methods description that adheres to the guidelines outlined in this report would be: "To minimize heterogeneity in genetic ancestry across our sample, we filtered our sample to only include individuals with a pairwise genotypic dissimilarity less than 10^{-3} to the centroid of the Yoruba of Ibadan sample of the 1000 Genomes Project." A possible critique of this language though is that this language may be perceived as bulky and difficult to apply throughout a study write-up. Researchers will be eager to find more concise language. In that regard, one possible approach is to favor using a sample abbreviation and the suffix *-like*. So, in a setting where conciseness is prioritized, instead of the above phrasing, one might say "1KG-YRI-like individuals" (see Box 5-3).

The overall approach of using an abbreviation and the *-like* suffix is compatible with other descriptors, such as geographic and ethnic descriptors. So, one might for example, if scientifically justified, conduct a study on "self-described ethnically Italian individuals sampled in Houston, Texas, who are 1KG-TSI-like" to refer to self-described individuals sampled from Houston, Texas, who were further filtered based on genetic similarity to the 1000 Genome Project sample of Tuscans of Italy (TSI) individuals.

The approach also offers researchers flexibility regarding the choice of reference panels and the scale at which they are analyzed. For example, while the committee generally recommends against continental-scale conceptualizations of human genetic variation, in the "chromosome painting" (e.g., local ancestry calling) approaches that are common in human genetics, continental-scale conceptualizations are prominent in many analysis pipelines. In such settings, it is still possible, and favorable, to use concise descriptors (e.g., "we partition the genome into tracts that are 1KG-EUR-like and 1KG-AFR-like") in place of using continental ancestry labels as is common practice (e.g., "we portioned the genome into European

---

BOX 5-3
Concise Language for Genetic Similarity:
The Abbreviation + -Like System

Because the language used to fully describe population descriptors in terms of genetic similarity may be cumbersome, it may be useful to adopt an approach that uses a sample abbreviation and the suffix *like*.

For example, one might use the abbreviation "1KG-YRI-like individuals" for "individuals with a pairwise genotypic dissimilarity less than 10^{-3} to the Yoruba of Ibadan sample of the 1000 Genomes Project."

The use of *-like* as a suffix is a form of abbreviation for a procedure of defining similarity. Although there is an element of vagueness, it is concise, and for readers who need to understand the exact procedure used for ascribing this designation, they should be able to find in a well-written methods section what the precise procedures and thresholds used were to define the term.

Abbreviations are often disfavored in science communication and writing, but in this setting, attempts to use more accessible wording such as *European ancestry* in place of precise language are so prone to misunderstanding and propagating misconceptions that use of such terms is often counterproductive. An abbreviation implicitly invites a reader to read deeper into the technical meaning of the abbreviation rather than proceed with preconceived notions. For example, if one does not immediately recognize "1KG-YRI" as indicating the 1000 Genomes Project Yoruba of Ibadan (YRI) reference panel, they need to read deeper in the methods and understand what is meant.

"superpopulation"[2] (EUR) ancestry tracts and African "superpopulation" (AFR) ancestry tracts"). The changed language is concise and more information rich while avoiding the implication of clear continental boundaries in human genetic variation. For admixed individuals themselves, a harmonious approach using the language of genetic similarity would be to refer to the best approximating reference group; for example, "1KG-PEL-like," and "1KG-PUR-like" are two among many possible genetic similarity descriptors of Latino populations, with PEL = Peruvian in Lima, Peru, and PUR = Puerto Rican in Puerto Rico.

While potentially difficult to read by novices, the use of abbreviations for precision and conciseness is in fact a key aspect of scientific language in many fields (e.g., chemistry and the abbreviations for the elements, though the committee notes the analogy is not exact as there are no fundamental elements with regards to genetic ancestry). Their use in many scientific

---

[2] For example, the 1000 Genomes Project uses a classification of five superpopulations: Africans (AFR), Admixed Americans (AMR), East Asians (EAS), Europeans (EUR), and South Asians (SAS).

fields is evidence that abbreviations are not an impediment to scientific communication and can foster a culture of concise reference to precisely defined entities. A potential caveat of this approach is that one study's definition of *XX-like* may be different from another group's because of varying definitions to define a threshold on similarity. Standardization for such genetic similarity procedures may be feasible, and would be fruitful to develop, especially as a fuller representation of human genetic variation is sampled by ongoing studies. Nonetheless, the abbreviation plus *-like* approach would have less vagueness than the current widespread use of such terms as *European genetic ancestry* and *African genetic ancestry*, where both the reference populations and the methods to ascribe an affiliation to European or African sources are unclear and make implicit assumptions about the time frame of interest.

As investigators grapple with these complex challenges, harmonization efforts will continue to take many forms. Importantly, given the multiuse nature of modern data sets, any future harmonization efforts must be meaningful in how they aggregate populations or harmonize labels, while remaining flexible to uses and studies. Further alignment across the field to implement the recommendations and best practices described in this report can go a long way toward enhancing harmonization of the use of population descriptors (see Chapter 6).

REFERENCES

1000 Genomes Project Consortium. 2015. A global reference for human genetic variation. *Nature* 526:68-74.

Atkinson, E. G., A. X. Maihofer, M. Kanai, A. R. Martin, K. J. Karczewski, M. L. Santoro, J. C. Ulirsch, Y. Kamatani, Y. Okada, H. K. Finucane, K. C. Koenen, C. M. Nievergelt, M. J. Daly, and B. M. Neale. 2021. Tractor uses local ancestry to enable inclusion of admixed individuals in GWAS and to boost power. *Nature Genetics* 53(2):195-204.

Batai, K., S. Hooker, and R. A. Kittles. 2021. Leveraging genetic ancestry to study health disparities. *American Journal of Physical Anthropology* 175(2):363-375.

Benmarhnia, T., A. Hajat, and J. S. Kaufman. 2021. Inferential challenges when assessing racial/ethnic health disparities in environmental research. *Environmental Health* 20(1):7.

Bergström, A., S. A. McCarthy, R. Hui, M. A. Almarri, Q. Ayub, P. Danecek, Y. Chen, S. Felkel, P. Hallast, J. Kamm, H. Blanché, J.-F. Deleuze, H. Cann, S. Mallick, D. Reich, M. S. Sandhu, P. Skoglund, A. Scally, Y. Xue, R. Durbin, and C. Tyler-Smith. 2020. Insights into human genetic variation and population history from 929 diverse genomes. *Science* 367(6484):eaay5012.

Cann, H. M., C. de Toma, L. Cazes, M.-F. Legrand, V. Morel, L. Piouffre, J. Bodmer, W. F. Bodmer, B. Bonne-Tamir, A. Cambon-Thomsen, Z. Chen, J. Chu, C. Carcassi, L. Contu, R. Du, L. Excoffier, G. B. Ferrara, J. S. Friedlaender, H. Groot, D. Gurwitz, T. Jenkins, R. J. Herrera, X. Huang, J. Kidd, K. K. Kidd, A. Langaney, A. A. Lin, S. Q. Mehdi, P. Parham, A. Piazza, M. P. Pistillo, Y. Qian, Q. Shu, J. Xu, S. Zhu, J. L. Weber, H. T. Greely, M. W. Feldman, G. Thomas, J. Dausset, and L. L. Cavalli-Sforza. 2002. A human genome diversity cell line panel. *Science* 296(5566):261-262.

Chakraborty, R., S. A. Read, and S. J. Vincent. 2020. Understanding myopia: Pathogenesis and mechanisms. In *Updates on myopia: A clinical perspective*, edited by M. Ang and T. Y. Wong. Singapore: Springer Singapore. Pp. 65-94.

Charles, B. A., D. Shriner, and C. N. Rotimi. 2014. Accounting for linkage disequilibrium in association analysis of diverse populations. *Genetic Epidemiology* 38(3):265-273.

Choi, S. W., T. S.-H. Mak, and P. F. O'Reilly. 2020. Tutorial: A guide to performing polygenic risk score analyses. *Nature Protocols* 15(9):2759-2772.

Claw, K. G., M. Z. Anderson, R. L. Begay, K. S. Tsosie, K. Fox, N. A. Garrison, A. C. Bader, J. Bardill, D. A. Bolnick, J. Brooks, A. Cordova, R. S. Malhi, N. Nakatsuka, A. Neller, J. A. Raff, J. Singson, K. TallBear, T. Vargas, J. M. Yracheta, and Summer internship for INdigenous peoples in Genomics (SING) Consortium. 2018. A framework for enhancing ethical genomic research with indigenous communities. *Nature Communications* 9(1):2957.

Coop, G. 2023. Genetic similarity versus genetic ancestry groups as sample descriptors in human genetics. *arXiv* (preprint).

Daly, B., and O. I. Olopade. 2015. A perfect storm: How tumor biology, genomics, and health care delivery patterns collide to create a racial survival disparity in breast cancer and proposed interventions for change. *CA: A Cancer Journal for Clinicians* 65(3):221-238.

Delorey, T. M., C. G. K. Ziegler, G. Heimberg, R. Normand, Y. Yang, Å. Segerstolpe, D. Abbondanza, S. J. Fleming, A. Subramanian, D. T. Montoro, K. A. Jagadeesh, K. K. Dey, P. Sen, M. Slyper, Y. H. Pita-Juárez, D. Phillips, J. Biermann, Z. Bloom-Ackermann, N. Barkas, A. Ganna, J. Gomez, J. C. Melms, I. Katsyv, E. Normandin, P. Naderi, Y. V. Popov, S. S. Raju, S. Niezen, L. T. Y. Tsai, K. J. Siddle, M. Sud, V. M. Tran, S. K. Vellarikkal, Y. Wang, L. Amir-Zilberstein, D. S. Atri, J. Beechem, O. R. Brook, J. Chen, P. Divakar, P. Dorceus, J. M. Engreitz, A. Essene, D. M. Fitzgerald, R. Fropf, S. Gazal, J. Gould, J. Grzyb, T. Harvey, J. Hecht, T. Hether, J. Jané-Valbuena, M. Leney-Greene, H. Ma, C. McCabe, D. E. McLoughlin, E. M. Miller, C. Muus, M. Niemi, R. Padera, L. Pan, D. Pant, C. Pe'Er, J. Pfiffner-Borges, C. J. Pinto, J. Plaisted, J. Reeves, M. Ross, M. Rudy, E. H. Rueckert, M. Siciliano, A. Sturm, E. Todres, A. Waghray, S. Warren, S. Zhang, D. R. Zollinger, L. Cosimi, R. M. Gupta, N. Hacohen, H. Hibshoosh, W. Hide, A. L. Price, J. Rajagopal, P. R. Tata, S. Riedel, G. Szabo, T. L. Tickle, P. T. Ellinor, D. Hung, P. C. Sabeti, R. Novak, R. Rogers, D. E. Ingber, Z. G. Jiang, D. Juric, M. Babadi, S. L. Farhi, B. Izar, J. R. Stone, I. S. Vlachos, I. H. Solomon, O. Ashenberg, C. B. M. Porter, B. Li, A. K. Shalek, A.-C. Villani, O. Rozenblatt-Rosen, and A. Regev. 2021. COVID-19 tissue atlases reveal SARS-CoV-2 pathology and cellular targets. *Nature* 595(7865):107-113.

Doiron, D., P. Burton, Y. Marcon, A. Gaye, B. H. Wolffenbuttel, M. Perola, R. P. Stolk, L. Foco, C. Minelli, M. Waldenberger, R. Holle, K. Kvaløy, H. L. Hillege, A.-M. Tassé, V. Ferretti, and I. Fortier. 2013. Data harmonization and federated analysis of population-based studies: The BioSHaRE project. *Emerging Themes in Epidemiology* 10(1):12.

Dolitsky, S., A. Mitra, S. Khan, E. Ashkinadze, and M. V. Sauer. 2020. Beyond the "Jewish panel": The importance of offering expanded carrier screening to the Ashkenazi Jewish population. *F&S Reports* 1(3):294-298.

Eisenmann, S., E. Bánffy, P. van Dommelen, K. P. Hofmann, J. Maran, I. Lazaridis, A. Mittnik, M. McCormick, J. Krause, D. Reich, and P. W. Stockhammer. 2018. Reconciling material cultures in archaeology with genetic data: The nomenclature of clusters emerging from archaeogenomic analysis. *Scientific Reports* 8:13003.

Falconer, D. S., and T. F. C. Mackay. 1996. *Introduction to quantitative genetics*. 4th ed. Essex, England: Addison Wesley Longman Limited.

GeM-HD Consortium (Genetic Modifiers of Huntington's Disease Consortium). 2015. Identification of genetic factors that modify clinical onset of Huntington's disease. *Cell* 162(3):516-526.

Giannakopoulou, O., K. Lin, X. Meng, M.-H. Su, P.-H. Kuo, R. E. Peterson, S. Awasthi, A. Moscati, J. R. I. Coleman, N. Bass, I. Y. Millwood, Y. Chen, Z. Chen, H.-C. Chen, M.-L. Lu, M.-C. Huang, C.-H. Chen, E. A. Stahl, R. J. F. Loos, N. Mullins, R. J. Ursano, R. C. Kessler, M. B. Stein, S. Sen, L. J. Scott, M. Burmeister, Y. Fang, J. Tyrrell, Y. Jiang, C. Tian, A. M. McIntosh, S. Ripke, E. C. Dunn, K. S. Kendler, R. G. Walters, C. M. Lewis, K. Kuchenbaecker, N. R. Wray, S. Ripke, M. Mattheisen, M. Trzaskowski, E. M. Byrne, A. Abdellaoui, M. J. Adams, E. Agerbo, T. M. Air, T. F. M. Andlauer, S.-A. Bacanu, M. Bækvad-Hansen, A. T. F. Beekman, T. B. Bigdeli, E. B. Binder, J. Bryois, H. N. Buttenschøn, J. Bybjerg-Grauholm, N. Cai, E. Castelao, J. H. Christensen, T.-K. Clarke, J. R. I. Coleman, L. Colodro-Conde, H. Coon, B. Couvy-Duchesne, N. Craddock, G. E. Crawford, G. Davies, I. J. Deary, F. Degenhardt, E. M. Derks, N. Direk, C. V. Dolan, E. C. Dunn, T. C. Eley, V. Escott-Price, F. F. H. Kiadeh, H. K. Finucane, J. C. Foo, A. J. Forstner, J. Frank, H. A. Gaspar, M. Gill, F. S. Goes, S. D. Gordon, J. Grove, L. S. Hall, C. S. Hansen, T. F. Hansen, S. Herms, I. B. Hickie, P. Hoffmann, G. Homuth, C. Horn, J.-J. Hottenga, D. M. Howard, D. M. Hougaard, M. Ising, R. Jansen, I. Jones, L. A. Jones, E. Jorgenson, J. A. Knowles, I. S. Kohane, J. Kraft, W. W. Kretzschmar, Z. Kutalik, Y. Li, P. A. Lind, J. J. Luykx, D. J. Macintyre, D. F. Mackinnon, R. M. Maier, W. Maier, J. Marchini, H. Mbarek, P. McGrath, P. McGuffin, S. E. Medland, D. Mehta, C. M. Middeldorp, E. Mihailov, Y. Milaneschi, L. Milani, F. M. Mondimore, G. W. Montgomery, S. Mostafavi, N. Mullins, M. Nauck, B. Ng, M. G. Nivard, D. R. Nyholt, P. F. O'Reilly, H. Oskarsson, M. J. Owen, J. N. Painter, C. B. Pedersen, M. G. Pedersen, R. E. Peterson, E. Pettersson, W. J. Peyrot, G. Pistis, D. Posthuma, J. A. Quiroz, P. Qvist, J. P. Rice, B. P. Riley, M. Rivera, S. S. Mirza, R. Schoevers, E. C. Schulte, L. Shen, J. Shi, S. I. Shyn, E. Sigurdsson, G. C. B. Sinnamon, J. H. Smit, D. J. Smith, H. Stefansson, S. Steinberg, F. Streit, J. Strohmaier, K. E. Tansey, H. Teismann, A. Teumer, W. Thompson, P. A. Thompson, T. E. Thorgeirsson, M. Traylor, J. Treutlein, V. Trubetskoy, A. G. Uitterlinden, D. Umbricht, S. Van Der Auwera, A. M. Van Hemert, A. Viktorin, P. M. Visscher, Y. Wang, B. T. Webb, S. M. Weinsheimer, J. Wellmann, G. Willemsen, S. H. Witt, Y. Wu, H. S. Xi, J. Yang, F. Zhang, V. Arolt, B. T. Baune, K. Berger, D. I. Boomsma, S. Cichon, U. Dannlowski, F. De Geus, J. R. Depaulo, E. Domenici, K. Domschke, T. Esko, H. J. Grabe, S. P. Hamilton, C. Hayward, A. C. Heath, K. S. Kendler, S. Kloiber, G. Lewis, Q. S. Li, S. Lucae, P. A. Madden, P. K. Magnusson, N. G. Martin, A. M. McIntosh, A. Metspalu, O. Mors, P. B. Mortensen, B. Müller-Myhsok, M. Nordentoft, M. M. Nöthen, M. C. O'Donovan, S. A. Paciga, N. L. Pedersen, B. W. Penninx, R. H. Perlis, D. J. Porteous, J. B. Potash, M. Preisig, M. Rietschel, C. Schaefer, T. G. Schulze, J. W. Smoller, K. Stefansson, H. Tiemeier, R. Uher, H. Völzke, M. M. Weissman, T. Werge, C. M. Lewis, D. F. Levinson, G. Breen, A. D. Børglum, P. F. Sullivan, M. Agee, S. Aslibekyan, A. Auton, E. Babalola, R. K. Bell, J. Bielenberg, K. Bryc, E. Bullis, B. Cameron, D. Coker, G. Cuellar Partida, D. Dhamija, S. Das, S. L. Elson, T. Filshtein, K. Fletez-Brant, P. Fontanillas, W. Freyman, P. M. Gandhi, K. Heilbron, B. Hicks, D. A. Hinds, K. E. Huber, E. M. Jewett, Y. Jiang, A. Kleinman, K. Kukar, V. Lane, K.-H. Lin, M. Lowe, M. K. Luff, J. C. McCreight, M. H. McIntyre, K. F. McManus, S. J. Micheletti, M. E. Moreno, J. L. Mountain, S. V. Mozaffari, P. Nandakumar, E. S. Noblin, J. O'Connell, A. A. Petrakovitz, G. D. Poznik, M. Schumacher, A. J. Shastri, J. F. Shelton, J. Shi, S. Shringarpure, C. Tian, V. Tran, J. Y. Tung, X. Wang, W. Wang, C. H. Weldon, P. Wilton, D. Avery, D. Bennett, Z. Bian, R. Boxall, F. Bragg, K. H. Chan, L. Chang, Y. Chang, B. Chen, J. Chen, J. Chen, N. Chen, N. Chen, X. Chen, Y. Chen, Z. Chen, L. Cheng, J. Clarke, R. Clarke, R. Collins, C. Dong, H. Du, R. Du, Z. Fairhurst-Hunter, L. Fan, S. Feng, Z. Fu, W. Gan, R. Gao, Y. Gao, P. Ge, S. Gilbert, W. Gong, Q. Gu, Y. Guo, Z. Guo, Z. Guo, A. Hacker, X. Han, P. Hariri, P. He, T. He, M. Hill, M. Holmes, C. Hou, W. Hou, C. Hu, R. Hu, X. Hu, Y. Hu, H. Hua, Y. Hua, Y. Huang, P. K. Im, A. Iona, Q. Jiang, J. Jin, M. Kakkoura, Q. Kang, C. Kartsonaki, R. Kerosi, L. Kong, J. Lan, G. Lancaster, F. Li, H. Li, J. Li, L. Li, M. Li, S. Li, Y. Li, Y. Li, Z. Li, K. Lin, L. Lingli, C. Liu, D. Liu, D. Liu, F. Liu, H. Liu, J. Liu, J. Liu, Y.

Liu, Y. Liu, H. Long, Y. Lu, G. Luo, J. Lv, S. Lv, L. Ma, E. Mao, J. McDonnell, F. Meng, J. Meng, I. Millwood, Q. Nie, F. Ning, D. Pan, R. Pan, Z. Pang, P. Pei, R. Peto, A. Pozarickij, Y. Qian, Y. Qin, C. Qu, X. Ren, P. Ryder, S. Sansome, D. Schmidt, P. Sherliker, R. Sohoni, B. Stevens, J. Su, H. Sun, Q. Sun, X. Sun, A. Tang, Z. Tang, R. Tao, X. Tian, I. Turnbull, R. Walters, M. Wan, C. Wang, C. Wang, H. Wang, J. Wang, L. Wang, P. Wang, T. Wang, S. Wang, S. Wang, X. Wang, L. Wei, M. Weng, N. Wright, M. Wu, X. Wu, S. Wu, K. Xie, Q. Xu, Q. Xu, X. Xu, S. Yan, L. Yang, X. Yang, J. Yang, P. Yao, L. Yin, B. Yu, C. Yu, M. Yu, Y. Zhai, H. Zhang, H. Zhang, J. Zhang, L. Zhang, N. Zhang, X. Zhang, X. Zhang, X. Zhang, X. Zhong, D. Z. Zhou, G. Zhou, J. Zhou, L. Zhou, W. Zhou, X. Zhou, Y. Zhou, and M. Zou. 2021. The genetic architecture of depression in individuals of east Asian ancestry. *JAMA Psychiatry* 78(11):1258-1269.

Gutenkunst, R. N., R. D. Hernandez, S. H. Williamson, and C. D. Bustamante. 2009. Inferring the joint demographic history of multiple populations from multidimensional SNP frequency data. *PLoS Genetics* 5(10):e1000695.

Hardeman, R. R., P. A. Homan, T. Chantarat, B. A. Davis, and T. H. Brown. 2022. Improving the measurement of structural racism to achieve antiracist health policy: Study examines measurement of structural racism to achieve antiracist health policy. *Health Affairs* 41(2):179-186.

Hirschhorn, J. N., and M. J. Daly. 2005. Genome-wide association studies for common diseases and complex traits. *Nature Reviews Genetics* 6(2):95-108.

Jimenez-Sanchez, M., F. Licitra, B. R. Underwood, and D. C. Rubinsztein. 2017. Huntington's disease: Mechanisms of pathogenesis and therapeutic strategies. *Cold Spring Harbor Perspectives in Medicine* 7(7).

Khan, A. T., S. M. Gogarten, C. P. McHugh, A. M. Stilp, T. Sofer, M. L. Bowers, Q. Wong, L. A. Cupples, B. Hidalgo, A. D. Johnson, M.-L. N. McDonald, S. T. McGarvey, M. R. G. Taylor, S. M. Fullerton, M. P. Conomos, and S. C. Nelson. 2022. Recommendations on the use and reporting of race, ethnicity, and ancestry in genetic research: Experiences from the NHLBI TOPMed program. *Cell Genomics* 2(8):100155.

Khera, A. V., M. Chaffin, K. G. Aragam, M. E. Haas, C. Roselli, S. H. Choi, P. Natarajan, E. S. Lander, S. A. Lubitz, P. T. Ellinor, and S. Kathiresan. 2018. Genome-wide polygenic scores for common diseases identify individuals with risk equivalent to monogenic mutations. *Nature Genetics* 50(9):1219-1224.

Kistka, Z. A.-F., L. Palomar, K. A. Lee, S. E. Boslaugh, M. F. Wangler, F. S. Cole, M. R. Debaun, and L. J. Muglia. 2007. Racial disparity in the frequency of recurrence of preterm birth. *American Journal of Obstetrics and Gynecology* 196(2):131.e1-131.e6.

Kittles, R. A., E. R. Santos, N. S. Oji-Njideka, and C. Bonilla. 2007. Race, skin color and genetic ancestry: Implications for biomedical research on health disparities. *Californian Journal of Health Promotion* 5(Special Issue):9-23.

Lee, S. S.-J., S. M. Fullerton, A. Saperstein, and J. K. Shim. 2019. Ethics of inclusion: Cultivate trust in precision medicine. *Science* 364(6444):941-942.

Lesko, C. R., L. P. Jacobson, K. N. Althoff, A. G. Abraham, S. J. Gange, R. D. Moore, S. Modur, and B. Lau. 2018. Collaborative, pooled and harmonized study designs for epidemiologic research: Challenges and opportunities. *International Journal of Epidemiology* 47(2):654-668.

Lewis, A. C. F., S. J. Molina, P. S. Appelbaum, B. Dauda, A. Di Rienzo, A. Fuentes, S. M. Fullerton, N. A. Garrison, N. Ghosh, E. M. Hammonds, D. S. Jones, E. E. Kenny, P. Kraft, S. S. Lee, M. Mauro, J. Novembre, A. Panofsky, M. Sohail, B. M. Neale, and D. S. Allen. 2022. Getting genetic ancestry right for science and society. *Science* 376(6590):250-252.

Li, J., and Q. Zhang. 2017. Insight into the molecular genetics of myopia. *Molecular Vision* 23:1048.

Mallick, S., H. Li, M. Lipson, I. Mathieson, M. Gymrek, F. Racimo, M. Zhao, N. Chennagiri, S. Nordenfelt, A. Tandon, P. Skoglund, I. Lazaridis, S. Sankararaman, Q. Fu, N. Rohland, G. Renaud, Y. Erlich, T. Willems, C. Gallo, J. P. Spence, Y. S. Song, G. Poletti, F. Balloux, G. van Driem, P. de Knijff, I. G. Romero, A. R. Jha, D. M. Behar, C. M. Bravi, C. Capelli, T. Hervig, A. Moreno-Estrada, O. L. Posukh, E. Balanovska, O. Balanovsky, S. Karachanak-Yankova, H. Sahakyan, D. Toncheva, L. Yepiskoposyan, C. Tyler-Smith, Y. Xue, M. S. Abdullah, A. Ruiz-Linares, C. M. Beall, A. Di Rienzo, C. Jeong, E. B. Starikovskaya, E. Metspalu, J. Parik, R. Villems, B. M. Henn, U. Hodoglugil, R. Mahley, A. Sajantila, G. Stamatoyannopoulos, J. T. Wee, R. Khusainova, E. Khusnutdinova, S. Litvinov, G. Ayodo, D. Comas, M. F. Hammer, T. Kivisild, W. Klitz, C. A. Winkler, D. Labuda, M. Bamshad, L. B. Jorde, S. A. Tishkoff, W. S. Watkins, M. Metspalu, S. Dryomov, R. Sukernik, L. Singh, K. Thangaraj, S. Pääbo, J. Kelso, N. Patterson, and D. Reich. 2016. The Simons Genome Diversity Project: 300 genomes from 142 diverse populations. *Nature* 538(7624):201-206.

Martin, A. R., M. Kanai, Y. Kamatani, Y. Okada, B. M. Neale, and M. J. Daly. 2019. Clinical use of current polygenic risk scores may exacerbate health disparities: A systematic literature review. *Pharmacogenomics* 18(16):1541-1550. *Nature Genetics* 51(4):584-591.

Martinez, R. A. M., N. Andrabi, A. N. Goodwin, R. E. Wilbur, N. R. Smith, and P. N. Zivich. 2023. Conceptualization, operationalization, and utilization of race and ethnicity in major epidemiology journals 1995–2018: A systematic review. *American Journal of Epidemiology* 192(3):483-496.

Mathieson, I., and A. Scally. 2020. What is ancestry? *PLoS Genetics* 16(3):e1008624.

Mavaddat, N., K. Michailidou, J. Dennis, M. Lush, L. Fachal, A. Lee, J. P. Tyrer, T.-H. Chen, Q. Wang, M. K. Bolla, X. Yang, M. A. Adank, T. Ahearn, K. Aittomäki, J. Allen, I. L. Andrulis, H. Anton-Culver, N. N. Antonenkova, V. Arndt, K. J. Aronson, P. L. Auer, P. Auvinen, M. Barrdahl, L. E. Beane Freeman, M. W. Beckmann, S. Behrens, J. Benitez, M. Bermisheva, L. Bernstein, C. Blomqvist, N. V. Bogdanova, S. E. Bojesen, B. Bonanni, A.-L. Børresen-Dale, H. Brauch, M. Bremer, H. Brenner, A. Brentnall, I. W. Brock, A. Brooks-Wilson, S. Y. Brucker, T. Brüning, B. Burwinkel, D. Campa, B. D. Carter, J. E. Castelao, S. J. Chanock, R. Chlebowski, H. Christiansen, C. L. Clarke, J. M. Collée, E. Cordina-Duverger, S. Cornelissen, F. J. Couch, A. Cox, S. S. Cross, K. Czene, M. B. Daly, P. Devilee, T. Dörk, I. dos-Santos-Silva, M. Dumont, L. Durcan, M. Dwek, D. M. Eccles, A. B. Ekici, A. H. Eliassen, C. Ellberg, C. Engel, M. Eriksson, D. G. Evans, P. A. Fasching, J. Figueroa, O. Fletcher, H. Flyger, A. Försti, L. Fritschi, M. Gabrielson, M. Gago-Dominguez, S. M. Gapstur, J. A. García-Sáenz, M. M. Gaudet, V. Georgoulias, G. G. Giles, I. R. Gilyazova, G. Glendon, M. S. Goldberg, D. E. Goldgar, A. González-Neira, G. I. Grenaker Alnæs, M. Grip, J. Gronwald, A. Grundy, P. Guénel, L. Haeberle, E. Hahnen, C. A. Haiman, N. Håkansson, U. Hamann, S. E. Hankinson, E. F. Harkness, S. N. Hart, W. He, A. Hein, J. Heyworth, P. Hillemanns, A. Hollestelle, M. J. Hooning, R. N. Hoover, J. L. Hopper, A. Howell, G. Huang, K. Humphreys, D. J. Hunter, M. Jakimovska, A. Jakubowska, W. Janni, E. M. John, N. Johnson, M. E. Jones, A. Jukkola-Vuorinen, A. Jung, R. Kaaks, K. Kaczmarek, V. Kataja, R. Keeman, M. J. Kerin, E. Khusnutdinova, J. I. Kiiski, J. A. Knight, Y.-D. Ko, V.-M. Kosma, V. Koutros, V. N. Kristensen, U. Krüger, T. Kühl, D. Lambrechts, L. Le Marchand, E. Lee, F. Lejbkowicz, J. Lilyquist, A. Lindblom, S. Lindström, J. Lissowska, W.-Y. Lo, S. Loibl, J. Long, J. Lubiński, M. P. Lux, R. J. MacInnis, T. Maishman, E. Makalic, I. Maleva Kostovska, A. Mannermaa, S. Manoukian, S. Margolin, J. W. M. Martens, M. E. Martinez, D. Mavroudis, C. McLean, A. Meindl, U. Menon, P. Middha, N. Miller, F. Moreno, A. M. Mulligan, C. Mulot, V. M. Muñoz-Garzon, S. L. Neuhausen, H. Nevanlinna, P. Neven, W. G. Newman, S. F. Nielsen, B. G. Nordestgaard, A. Norman, K. Offit, J. E. Olson, H. Olsson, N. Orr, V. S. Pankratz, T.-W. Park-Simon, J. I. A. Perez, C. Pérez-Barrios, P. Peterlongo, J. Peto, M. Pinchev, D. Plaseska-Karanfilska, E. C. Polley, R. Prentice, N. Presneau, D. Prokofyeva, K. Purrington, K. Pylkäs, B. Rack, P. Radice, R.

Rau-Murthy, G. Rennert, H. S. Rennert, V. Rhenius, M. Robson, A. Romero, K. J. Ruddy, M. Ruebner, E. Saloustros, D. P. Sandler, E. J. Sawyer, D. F. Schmidt, R. K. Schmutzler, A. Schneeweiss, M. J. Schoemaker, F. Schumacher, P. Schürmann, L. Schwentner, C. Scott, R. J. Scott, C. Seynaeve, M. Shah, M. E. Sherman, M. J. Shrubsole, X.-O. Shu, S. Slager, A. Smeets, C. Sohn, P. Soucy, M. C. Southey, J. J. Spinelli, C. Stegmaier, J. Stone, A. J. Swerdlow, R. M. Tamimi, W. J. Tapper, J. A. Taylor, M. B. Terry, K. Thöne, R. A. E. M. Tollenaar, I. Tomlinson, T. Truong, M. Tzardi, H.-U. Ulmer, M. Untch, C. M. Vachon, E. M. van Veen, J. Vijai, C. R. Weinberg, C. Wendt, A. S. Whittemore, H. Wildiers, W. Willett, R. Winqvist, A. Wolk, X. R. Yang, D. Yannoukakos, Y. Zhang, W. Zheng, A. Ziogas, A. M. Dunning, D. J. Thompson, G. Chenevix-Trench, J. Chang-Claude, M. K. Schmidt, P. Hall, R. L. Milne, P. D. P. Pharoah, A. C. Antoniou, N. Chatterjee, P. Kraft, M. García-Closas, J. Simard, and D. F. Easton. 2019. Polygenic risk scores for prediction of breast cancer and breast cancer subtypes. *American Journal of Human Genetics* 104(1):21-34.

Mills, M. C., and C. Rahal. 2020. The GWAS diversity monitor tracks diversity by disease in real time. *Nature Genetics* 52(3):242-243.

Mostafavi, H., A. Harpak, I. Agarwal, D. Conley, J. K. Pritchard, and M. Przeworski. 2020. Variable prediction accuracy of polygenic scores within an ancestry group. *eLife* 9:e48376.

NASEM (National Academies of Sciences, Engineering, and Medicine). 2019. *Reproducibility and replicability in science*. Washington, DC: The National Academies Press.

Nazareth, S. B., G. A. Lazarin, and J. D. Goldberg. 2015. Changing trends in carrier screening for genetic disease in the United States. *Prenatal Diagnosis* 35(10):931-935.

Nielsen, R., J. M. Akey, M. Jakobsson, J. K. Pritchard, S. Tishkoff, and E. Willerslev. 2017. Tracing the peopling of the world through genomics. *Nature* 541:302-310.

O'Neal, W. K., and M. R. Knowles. 2018. Cystic fibrosis disease modifiers: Complex genetics defines the phenotypic diversity in a monogenic disease. *Annual Review of Genomics and Human Genetics* 19:201-222.

Okbay, A., Y. Wu, N. Wang, H. Jayashankar, M. Bennett, S. M. Nehzati, J. Sidorenko, H. Kweon, G. Goldman, T. Gjorgjieva, Y. Jiang, B. Hicks, C. Tian, D. A. Hinds, R. Ahlskog, P. K. E. Magnusson, S. Oskarsson, C. Hayward, A. Campbell, D. J. Porteous, J. Freese, P. Herd, 23andMe Research Team, Social Science Genetic Association Consortium, C. Watson, J. Jala, D. Conley, P. D. Koellinger, M. Johannesson, D. Laibson, M. N. Meyer, J. J. Lee, A. Kong, L. Yengo, D. Cesarini, P. Turley, P. M. Visscher, J. P. Beauchamp, D. J. Benjamin, and A. I. Young. 2022. Polygenic prediction of educational attainment within and between families from genome-wide association analyses in 3 million individuals. *Nature Genetics* 54(4):437-449.

Oni-Orisan, A., Y. Mavura, Y. Banda, T. A. Thornton, and R. Sebro. 2021. Embracing genetic diversity to improve black health. *New England Journal of Medicine* 384(12):1163-1167.

Parra, E. J., R. A. Kittles, and M. D. Shriver. 2004. Implications of correlations between skin color and genetic ancestry for biomedical research. *Nature Genetics* 36(S11):S54-S60.

Patterson, N., P. Moorjani, Y. Luo, S. Mallick, N. Rohland, Y. Zhan, T. Genschoreck, T. Webster, and D. Reich. 2012. Ancient admixture in human history. *Genetics* 192(3):1065-1093.

Pavličev, M., and G. P. Wagner. 2022. The value of broad taxonomic comparisons in evolutionary medicine: Disease is not a trait but a *state of a trait*! *MedComm* 3(4):e174.

Pritchard, J. K., M. Stephens, and P. Donnelly. 2000. Inference of population structure using multilocus genotype data. *Genetics* 155(2):945-959.

Privé, F., H. Aschard, S. Carmi, L. Folkersen, C. Hoggart, P. F. O'Reilly, and B. J. Vilhjálmsson. 2022. Portability of 245 polygenic scores when derived from the UK Biobank and applied to 9 ancestry groups from the same cohort. *American Journal of Human Genetics* 109(1):12-23.

Randolph, H. E., J. K. Fiege, B. K. Thielen, C. K. Mickelson, M. Shiratori, J. Barroso-Batista, R. A. Langlois, and L. Barreiro. 2021. Genetic ancestry effects on the response to viral infection are pervasive but cell type specific. *Science* 374(6571):1127-1133.

Rohde, D. L. T., S. Olson, and J. T. Chang. 2004. Modelling the recent common ancestry of all living humans. *Nature* 431(7008):562-566.

Sadarangani, M., A. Marchant, and T. R. Kollmann. 2021. Immunological mechanisms of vaccine-induced protection against COVID-19 in humans. *Nature Reviews Immunology* 21(8):475-484.

Schaefer, N. K., B. Shapiro, and R. E. Green. 2021. An ancestral recombination graph of human, Neanderthal, and Denisovan genomes. *Science Advances* 7(29):eabc0776.

Scheinfeldt, L. B., S. Soi, C. Lambert, W.-Y. Ko, A. Coulibaly, A. Ranciaro, S. Thompson, J. Hirbo, W. Beggs, M. Ibrahim, T. Nyambo, S. Omar, D. Woldemeskel, G. Belay, A. Froment, J. Kim, and S. A. Tishkoff. 2019. Genomic evidence for shared common ancestry of east African hunting-gathering populations and insights into local adaptation. *Proceedings of the National Academy of Sciences* 116(10):4166-4175.

Scutari, M., I. Mackay, and D. Balding. 2016. Using genetic distance to infer the accuracy of genomic prediction. *PLoS Genetics* 12(9):e1006288.

Shriner, D. 2013. Overview of admixture mapping. *Current Protocols in Human Genetics* Chapter 1:Unit 1.23.

Simons, C., N. I. Wolf, N. McNeil, L. Caldovic, J. M. Devaney, A. Takanohashi, J. Crawford, K. Ru, S. M. Grimmond, D. Miller, D. Tonduti, J. L. Schmidt, R. S. Chudnow, R. van Coster, L. Lagae, J. Kisler, J. Sperner, M. S. van der Knaap, R. Schiffmann, R. J. Taft, and A. Vanderver. 2013. A de novo mutation in the beta-tubulin gene TUBB4A results in the leukoencephalopathy hypomyelination with atrophy of the basal ganglia and cerebellum. *American Journal of Human Genetics* 92(5):767-773.

Sirugo, G., S. M. Williams, and S. A. Tishkoff. 2019. The missing diversity in human genetic studies. *Cell* 177(1):26-31.

Spratt, D. E., T. Chan, L. Waldron, C. Speers, F. Y. Feng, O. O. Ogunwobi, and J. R. Osborne. 2016. Racial/ethnic disparities in genomic sequencing. *JAMA Oncology* 2(8):1070.

Tan, T. Y., O. J. Dillon, Z. Stark, D. Schofield, K. Alam, R. Shrestha, B. Chong, D. Phelan, G. R. Brett, E. Creed, A. Jarmolowicz, P. Yap, M. Walsh, L. Downie, D. J. Amor, R. Savarirayan, G. McGillivray, A. Yeung, H. Peters, S. J. Robertson, A. J. Robinson, I. Macciocca, S. Sadedin, K. Bell, A. Oshlack, P. Georgeson, N. Thorne, C. Gaff, and S. M. White. 2017. Diagnostic impact and cost-effectiveness of whole-exome sequencing for ambulant children with suspected monogenic conditions. *JAMA Pediatrics* 171(9):855-862.

Teteh, D. K., L. Dawkins-Moultin, S. Hooker, W. Hernandez, C. Bonilla, D. Galloway, V. LaGroon, E. R. Santos, M. Shriver, C. D. M. Royal, and R. A. Kittles. 2020. Genetic ancestry, skin color and social attainment: The four cities study. *PLoS ONE* 15(8):e0237041.

Thornton, T. A., and J. L. Bermejo. 2014. Local and global ancestry inference and applications to genetic association analysis for admixed populations. *Genetic Epidemiology* 38(S1):S5-S12.

Torkamani, A., N. E. Wineinger, and E. J. Topol. 2018. The personal and clinical utility of polygenic risk scores. *Nature Reviews Genetics* 19(9):581-590.

Torres, J. B., and R. A. Kittles. 2007. The relationship between "race" and genetics and biomedical research. *Current Hypertension Reports* 9(3):196-201.

Turner, T. N., B. P. Coe, D. E. Dickel, K. Hoekzema, B. J. Nelson, M. C. Zody, Z. N. Kronenberg, F. Hormozdiari, A. Raja, L. A. Pennacchio, R. B. Darnell, and E. E. Eichler. 2017. Genomic patterns of de novo mutation in simplex autism. *Cell* 171(3):710-722.e712.

Van Alten, S., B. W. Domingue, T. Galama, and A. T. Marees. 2022. Reweighting the UK Biobank to reflect its underlying sampling population substantially reduces pervasive selection bias due to volunteering. *medRxiv* (preprint).

Visscher, P. M., N. R. Wray, Q. Zhang, P. Sklar, M. I. McCarthy, M. A. Brown, and J. Yang. 2017. 10 years of GWAS discovery: Biology, function, and translation. *American Journal of Human Genetics* 101(1):5-22.

Wallace, S. E., E. Kirby, and B. M. Knoppers. 2020. How can we not waste legacy genomic research data? *Frontiers in Genetics* 11:446.

Wang, Y., J. Guo, G. Ni, J. Yang, P. M. Visscher, and L. Yengo. 2020. Theoretical and empirical quantification of the accuracy of polygenic scores in ancestry divergent populations. *Nature Communications* 11(1).

Wang, Y., K. Tsuo, M. Kanai, B. M. Neale, and A. R. Martin. 2022. Challenges and opportunities for developing more generalizable polygenic risk scores. *Annual Review of Biomedical Data Science* 5:293-320.

Wexler, N. S. 2004. Venezuelan kindreds reveal that genetic and environmental factors modulate Huntington's disease age of onset. *Proceedings of the National Academy of Sciences* 101(10):3498-3503.

6

Implementation and Accountability

[This] conversation has been going on for a long time without much reso-lution—that suggests that perhaps we're asking the wrong question or that there are some important structural barriers in the practices of science that have prevented us from making progress. Standardization of population descriptors is a misguided goal. It creates a false sense of comparability across data sets, and it might actually also be disrespectful to participants. Instead of standardization of population descriptors, I think we ought to spend much more time in our genome science collecting data about culture, social experience, social status, and environmental exposures. I think if we have good measures of those things, we're much more likely to have replicable genome science.

—Pilar Ossorio, testimony to the committee
in a public session on April 4, 2022

INTRODUCTION

As was noted in Chapter 1, this is not the first report, publication, or conference proceedings to recommend ways to change how descent-associated population descriptors should be used in genetics and genomics. Nor should it be the final word in an evolving field. There are a few elements, though, that make this report distinct. One is the political climate in which it is proffered. In the time following the historic social events of 2020, there has arisen an urgency in research and health care institutions to examine, address, and change the structural racism that is embedded in many systems (Bailey et al., 2020; Churchwell et al., 2020). Another is the committee's attempt to examine the entire research ecosystem, from funders, researchers, and their institutions to study participants, journals, and professional societies. A third defining feature of the report is the subject of this chapter. The committee strongly believes that for this report to change both individual and collective behavior, the recommendations need to be actionable, the implementation processes should contain incentives, and the people and institutions involved need to be held accountable on an ongoing basis and in meaningful ways to demonstrate progress toward specific goals.

IMPLEMENTATION ACROSS THE GENOMICS RESEARCH ECOSYSTEM

There are many players in the genomics research ecosystem. To make the changes recommended in this report, there is a need for partnership among all of these interested parties to support the researchers during this process of implementation; working together across the research enterprise offers part of the solution. Moreover, there is a shared responsibility for making these changes across an interdisciplinary research community. Without support for these changes throughout the community, the burden of implementation will likely fall disproportionately on individual researchers, who typically lack the personnel and funding resources to adhere to noncompulsory guidelines in a sustainable fashion.

The recommendations and the strategies to implement them presented in Chapters 4 and 5 are directed primarily to researchers. In this chapter, the focus is on the other relevant parties who are equally responsible in effecting lasting change in how population descriptors are used in genetics and genomics research. It will be evident that all of these recommendations and strategies also involve or affect research scientists. To fully implement these recommendations as well as create structures and systems that enable and incentivize researchers to collect and include environmental data and engage communities, support from institutions and funding agencies is needed to facilitate collaborations between genetics researchers and researchers in other disciplines such as the social sciences.

Study Participants and their Communities

While study participants are essential to a research project probing human genetics or genomics, these individuals or communities typically have little say in how their data are used and reported, though that is changing with platforms such as LunaDNA[1] and Genetic Alliance Registry[2] that place people at the center of the decision making about when and how their

---

[1] https://www.lunadna.com/ (accessed January 3, 2023).
[2] https://geneticalliance.org/registries/ga-registry (accessed January 3, 2023).

health information is used. Traditionally, individual study participants often are given a limited list of population labels to choose from, and these often fail to capture how they identify themselves (Kaplan and Bennett, 2003), as evidenced by the increase in the checking of the "some other race" box or of multiple boxes in the current census categories (Roman, 2022). Moreover, research staff responsible for recruitment may guess or assume population labels for the study participants (Borrell et al., 2021) to avoid having missing data. And even if participants self-identify to their own satisfaction, researchers may later combine them into categories with labels that no longer capture the identity that participants would have selected themselves (Hunt and Megyesi, 2008). These issues violate the guiding principles of *respect, beneficence,* and *equity and justice* (see Chapter 3).

To improve this misalignment of identities, researchers working in close partnership with individual study participants, and especially communities, can work to better understand how individuals identify themselves and, in some cases, why these are the descriptors or group labels they will use. When individuals are empowered to identify themselves on their terms, and have input into the research study design, they are more likely to have trust and investment in the study and its outcomes (CTSA Consortium, 2011). A more person-centered model is adopted in some community-based studies investigating population genetics, because in these studies, getting to know the community is already understood and accepted as a necessary prerequisite to collecting data. Without this partnership, some communities may refuse to participate, as they have in the past. A person-centered model is not typically the case in larger studies (e.g., long-term studies of health and disease) and becomes especially problematic when data from multiple studies, often collected at different times, are merged for analysis. It should be noted that community engagement may add additional costs as well as burden to participants and the community, specifically of their time, which could reduce participation by diverse communities.

In some situations, though, researchers may have to limit the number of population categories they can use for their study in order to have groups that are large enough to yield statistically robust answers, or to properly address a specific question within the study with adequate statistical power (IOM, 2009). In these cases, consent should be sought to aggregate individuals in particular ways, with a dialogue between researchers and participants as to why it may involve altering their population identities. Clear information should be provided to study participants about the study design, methods, objectives, and possible outcomes and impact. This information should be supplied by the researchers or, perhaps in larger studies, by the funding agency. Respect for participants can also be evoked by recognizing and including mechanisms in a study for nondisclosure of data as well as the possibility for participants to exit the study or revoke consent.

Conclusion 6-1. Forging partnerships between researchers and study participants and their communities is critically important and has benefits beyond building trust and mutual respect between relevant parties. By working collaboratively with study participants, researchers will better understand the identities, cultures, traditions, and practices of communities, thus improving the understanding of the types of information that should and could be collected for a strong study where the outcomes could, in turn, have the ability to improve the health of the communities who participate.

Funders of Genetics and Genomics Research

Funding agencies and organizations can play a major role in changing how population descriptors are used. For example, they could establish requirements to follow the recommendations in this report for all funding requests, reviews, and decisions. When developing funding concepts, requests for information or proposals could promote the recommendations and encourage adherence to them. One tool to assist researchers as they prepare their proposals would be a checklist, such as the Preferred Reporting Items for Systematic Review and Meta-Analyses (PRISMA),[3] Consolidated criteria for Reporting Qualitative research (COREQ),[4] and Consolidated Standards of Reporting Trials (CONSORT)[5] checklists used for systematic reviews, qualitative research, and clinical trials, respectively. A simple and clear checklist can be a useful tool for changing behavior and being proactive about avoiding commonly made errors (e.g., World Health Organization (WHO) surgical safety checklist).[6] A sample of what a checklist might contain for researchers using population descriptors in genetics research is in Box 6-1. As with other checklists, the intent is to make clear to researchers at the beginning of the study development or application process what they need to include. It promotes transparency and enables researchers to carefully evaluate the role and need for specific population descriptors in their proposal. A variation of the checklist is a decision tree, another tool for assisting the researcher in evaluating whether to use population descriptors, and if so, which ones are appropriate to use based on the objectives of their research and the characteristics of their data, among other features (see Appendix D and Chapter 5 for more detail). A checklist or decision tree

---

[3] https://prisma-statement.org/prismastatement/Checklist.aspx (accessed January 3, 2023).

[4] https://cdn.elsevier.com/promis_misc/ISSM_COREQ_Checklist.pdf (accessed January 3, 2023).

[5] https://www.consort-statement.org/media/default/downloads/CONSORT%202010%20 Checklist.pdf (accessed January 3, 2023).

[6] https://www.who.int/teams/integrated-health-services/patient-safety/research/safe-surgery/ tool-and-resources (accessed January 3, 2023).

BOX 6-1
Example Checklist that Funders of
Genetics and Genomics Research Can Implement for
Researchers

- What is the source of the data for your study?
- Are these individual-level data or group-level summary data?
- Have you clearly defined the purpose of your study?
- Have you engaged with the community that you would like to study?
- Has the community that is offering the use of their data to you had opportunities to identify themselves and explain why these are the descriptors they use to identify themselves? (Alternatively, has the research group sharing data provided guidance for how to develop population descriptors for the communities they have sampled?)
- Has consent been given for broad reuse of the data in research?
- Have you completed any required training on population descriptors?
- Have you determined which population descriptors are most appropriate for your study and understand why?
- Is interdisciplinary expertise needed to design and conduct the study and evaluate the data?
- Do you have a plan to clearly communicate the results of your study with the research community, including research participants?
- Do you plan to collect multiple descriptors, including specific measures of relevant environmental factors?

---

supports the guiding principles of *validity*, *reproducibility*, and *replicability* (see Chapter 3).

Funding agencies can further support this report's recommendations during the review of grant applications. For example, currently, researchers are not required to explain why a certain category of population descriptors was chosen and how they will be treated in statistical analysis, nor is this systematically evaluated in the study section. Desirable change would be greatly motivated if a study section were to consider how researchers intend to use population descriptors during the procedural checks for human research protocols. To assist both researchers and reviewers, a table or form would permit a more objective determination as to whether a proposal has addressed the necessary issues around using and reporting population descriptors and can be equally applied across all proposals. A similar form could assist in the poststudy reporting process, since many times the anticipated labels may change depending on the sample composition and how individuals self-identify.

One of the challenges for researchers in adopting the report's recommendations is that the Office of Management and Budget (OMB) Directive

15 has confounded the way that population descriptors are used and reported in genetics and genomics research (see the section "Population Classification Schemes in Genetics and Genomics Research" in Chapter 1).

> *Conclusion 6-2. It would be a helpful step in implementing this report's recommendations if funding agencies instructed researchers that they do not have to use the OMB categories to group individuals in their scientific work. Researchers need to know that, in general, they only have to use these categories when reporting study participant demographics of those they recruited. That is, the need and rationale for reporting to funding agencies is distinct from how researchers design their study and analyze their data. In the latter cases, researchers should use the most appropriate population descriptors for the questions they are probing instead of using the OMB categories reflexively.*

Professional Societies and Research Journals

Over the past several decades, a number of professional societies have developed statements or guidelines on race, ethnicity, human diversity, and multicultural practices. Statements, such as the one on race published by the American Association of Physical Anthropologists (AAPA, 1996), were intended for their members and colleagues and not specifically focused on genetics. During the Office of Management and Budget's review of Directive 15, the American Anthropological Association (AAA) submitted a set of recommendations in response to the OMB–requested comment period for the recommendations from the Interagency Committee (AAA, 1997) based on the similar scientific thinking espoused by the AAPA the previous year. The next year, the AAA prepared a statement on race for its members (AAA, 1998). Twenty years ago, the American Psychological Association (APA) prepared an extensive set of guidelines intended to assist their members and fellow psychologists in improving their cross-cultural interactions (APA, 2003). Recognizing that the concepts of race, ethnicity, and culture are dynamic, several of these societies have updated their guidelines recently (APA, 2017, 2019; Fuentes et al., 2019). Other organizations, like the American Medical Association (AMA), have followed suit (AMA, 2020a,b).

In every case, the guidelines have been aspirational and intended to encourage their professional colleagues to become educated and informed about how they view race, ethnicity, ancestry, and other descriptors, and to be aware of how they use these descriptors and associated language in their research, practice, writing, and conversation. For example, the AMA recommends "that clinicians and researchers focus on genetics and biology, the experience of racism, and social determinants of health when describing risk factors for disease" (AMA, 2020b). However, these factors are conflated.

In some cases, the guidelines of a professional society inform the guidelines or standards of their journals. For example, *American Psychologist*, the APA's flagship journal, requires authors to use "bias-free and community-driven language" (APA, 2022), which is explained in the *APA Publication Manual*. *Genetics in Medicine*, which is an official journal of the American College of Medical Genetics and Genomics, provides author guidelines for reporting on diversity, race, ethnicity, sex, and gender.[7] Likewise, the *Journal of the American Medical Association (JAMA)* has detailed guidance on reporting on race and ethnicity (Flanagin et al., 2021). *JAMA*'s guidelines have been adopted by other publications, such as the *American Journal of Human Genetics* (B. Korf, AJHG, personal communication, September 16, 2022).

The difficulty these societies and their journals face is how to get members and authors to abide by these guidelines. Journals can require that certain types of language be used or avoided, and they can memorialize that in their style guides and have their editors enforce the standards (e.g., *Nature Human Behavior*)[8] (Flanagin et al., 2021). But this is insufficient. What is necessary is an understanding of the underlying issues during study design and long before data analyses: the moment of publication is far too late.

As was suggested to funding agencies to facilitate the submission of grant applications, journals could create a checklist focused on population descriptors and how researchers should present them in the methods and results sections, in tables and figures, and what explanatory information is needed concerning why certain descriptors were chosen for or left out of an analysis (for example, see Box 6-2). Journals could come together to adopt the principles and recommendations in this report through organizations that are set up to change the publishing culture such as the Committee on Publication Ethics. This committee provides both best practices and education modules to set a new standard for adopting ethical publishing practices across a variety of disciplines internationally.

Among their other uses, publications are an essential measure of a researcher's productivity. As such, "getting published" can be a powerful incentive, so journal editors have leverage that could encourage researchers, and perhaps other entities within the research ecosystem such as research institutions, to change how they understand and use descent-associated population descriptors. For example, a journal could adopt the recommendations in this report by creating editorial review checks to ensure that authors whose papers are sent out for peer review have adhered to these recommendations.

---

[7] https://www.elsevier.com/journals/genetics-in-medicine/1098-3600/guide-for-authors (accessed January 3, 2023).

[8] https://www.nature.com/nathumbehav/editorial-policies/ethics-and-biosecurity#race-ethnicity-racism (accessed January 3, 2023).

BOX 6-2
Example Checklist that Journals Can Implement for Genomics Researchers

- Is there a description in the methods section of population descriptors (e.g., race and/or ethnicity, geography) that were collected?
- Are the source data of each population descriptor reported (e.g., database, electronic health record, survey)?
- Is there a description of how participant population descriptors were selected and how group labels were assigned?
- Is a scientific justification provided for collection of population descriptor data?
- Are population descriptors being used as proxies for environmental variables? If so, is this noted and explained?
- Are appropriate reference categories for the populations of interest being used as reference categories in analysis? Is there a scientific justification for these approaches?
- In studies of genetic contributions to health disparities, are social influences, environmental exposures, and other likely relevant variables included? If not, is the lack of assessment of the possible roles of these nongenetic factors discussed as a limitation?

SOURCE: Adapted from *Genetics in Medicine*'s Guide for Authors, https://www.elsevier.com/journals/genetics-in-medicine/1098-3600/guide-for-authors.

Research Institutions

The climate and infrastructure of research institutions greatly influence the ways in which research is carried out within their organizations. Thus, universities, private research centers, and government agencies are key partners in assisting researchers as they strive to implement this report's recommendations and adhere to its guiding principles.

This report was created by an interdisciplinary team of geneticists and social scientists. This combination of expertise and points of view has been essential in developing the recommendations, guiding principles, and strategies for implementation. The committee feels strongly that research in human genetics and genomics would benefit from collaborations between social scientists (such as anthropologists, sociologists, and demographers), historians, ethicists, epidemiologists, and biologists. Institutions can facilitate these interactions through the development of infrastructure that makes collaborations easy to start, supporting them financially, and encouraging researchers to form and sustain collaborations. There are several examples that could serve as models: Northwestern University's Institute for Policy

Research's Cells to Society–The Center on Social Disparities and Health[9]; UCLA's Institute for Society and Genetics[10]; Duke University's Office of Interdisciplinary Studies[11]; and University of Wisconsin-Madison's Center for Demography of Health and Aging,[12] to name a few.

One of the confounding issues in studying trait variation is distinguishing between genetic and environmental factors (see Chapter 2). Geneticists focus on understanding the causes and consequences of human genetic variation. Factors that interfere with accurately determining these effects create barriers to optimal genetics research that may be addressed through study design and analysis. Geneticists and researchers using genetic and genomic tools may lack the social and environmental data they need to analyze the most appropriate nongenetic variables. They may also lack the training and expertise to design and carry out a study that will collect those data. Collaborations among geneticists, epidemiologists, demographers, and other social scientists can therefore improve study design and statistical analysis of the data to better differentiate between genetic and nongenetic factors and their effects.

Researchers, from undergraduate students to principal investigators, could benefit from continuing education on the bias and misuse of population descriptors in scientific and medical research. New York University (NYU), for example, developed a workshop in 2021 called Race and Racism in the Sciences, hosted by the departments of biology and psychology and the NYU Center for Neural Science.[13] It is compulsory for some graduate students and strongly recommended for all other members of these three communities. Funding agencies could collaborate with research institutions on developing and holding training and continuing education about the proper use of population descriptors.

In addition, researchers could be required to complete training about the use of population descriptors before engaging in research with human participants and before being granted access to data sets. NIH's *All of Us* Research Program requires training on "responsible and ethical research" prior to using the Researcher Workbench (All of Us, 2022). These trainings could contain information about the labels that are used within the data set, explaining how they can or cannot be used within research projects using the data set.

---

[9] https://www.ipr.northwestern.edu/what-we-study/social-disparities-and-health/ (accessed January 3, 2023).

[10] https://socgen.ucla.edu/ (accessed January 3, 2023).

[11] https://sites.duke.edu/interdisciplinary/ (accessed January 3, 2023).

[12] https://cdha.wisc.edu/ (accessed January 3, 2023).

[13] https://as.nyu.edu/departments/cns/events/EventDescriptions/WorkshopRace.html (accessed January 3, 2023).

The committee encourages the development of computational tools able to compare studies and identify differences in the metadata related to population descriptors. The tools could then assist a researcher in deciding whether merging the data sets would corrupt the metadata and enable them to use the merged data to address a question of interest. In addition, research on frameworks for the development and dissemination of genetic data resources, such as allele frequencies, should prioritize the use of genetic similarity, rather than other population descriptors (race, ethnicity, geography), which may be poor proxies for genetic backgrounds that form the basis of these groupings. The committee hopes that educating investigators on the use of population descriptors will facilitate the development of these computational and other methodological tools.

Journalists, Media, and Researchers: An Important Partnership for Clearly Communicating Research Findings

Sometimes scientific findings create new knowledge that is relevant not only to specialized audiences but also to the general population. Conveying that information accurately and effectively to the lay public is the purview of science journalists and other science communication specialists. As the genomics research ecosystem evolves in how it uses descent-associated population descriptors, and as genetics and genomics research advances common understanding of human health and disease and becomes more popular, partnerships between science journalists and basic and clinical scientists will be ever more important. One way to facilitate this partnership is for the press offices of research institutions to receive training on best practices for the use of population descriptors, since it is typically the people in these offices who interact directly with scientists to translate their research findings and technical terminology into language that is understandable by the general public while retaining the accuracy and nuances of the science. In addition, researchers should be trained to produce easily understandable summaries of their research findings that properly convey the subtleties of using population descriptors in genomics research. These summaries could be provided to newspaper and other popular media reporters when they write about relevant research findings (Takezawa et al., 2014).

For this report to reach full penetrance in society and for its recommendations to have a lasting effect, what this committee has written will need to weave its way into the general consciousness alongside the many other conversations about diversity, inclusion, equity, and justice. It would thus be beneficial if journalists and reporters became familiar with both this report's main messages and the committee's rationale for its decisions. Broadly disseminating this report's messages through their many different media outlets will be a powerful way to effect change and drive implementation of the committee's recommendations.

RECOMMENDATIONS

The effectiveness of the following recommendations in advancing trust in and improving the quality of results from genomics research will depend upon how they are implemented. Many aspects of the current systems that fund, support, evaluate, and reward genomics research may impede rather than facilitate their implementation. Changing these systems will, over time, lead to more effective implementation of these recommendations.

Funding agencies, research institutions (including associated institutional review boards and other activities with research participants), research journals, professional societies, and lay media professionals should evaluate their processes and structures related to the use of population descriptors in genomics research and report to their communities whether or not they are facilitating the recommendations in this report. A plan should be provided, along with a timeline, to change processes and structures that are not aligned with these recommendations. If processes and structures cannot be changed, this should be made transparent, along with a justification as to why the changes cannot be made and how this misalignment will be mitigated in the context of this committee's report recommendations.

> Recommendation 9. Funding agencies, research institutions, research journals, and professional societies should offer tools widely to their communities to facilitate the implementation of these recommendations; these tools should be publicly available, especially when they are supported by public funds. Such tools could include:
> - educational modules for inclusion in human research protection training[14];
> - manuscript submission and review guidelines;
> - grant submission and review criteria;
> - training and education of trainees at all levels;
> - opportunities for continuing education for researchers; and
> - informatics tools, such as data structure standards for sharing labels and labeling procedures used within a study.

> Recommendation 10. Research institutions and funding agencies should embed incentives for fostering interdisciplinary collaboration among researchers with different areas of expertise, including genetics and ge-

---

[14] Often called "human subjects" research training. See also https://www.hhs.gov/ohrp/education-and-outreach/human-research-protection-training/index.html (accessed January 3, 2023).

nomics, social sciences, epidemiology, and community-based research, to facilitate the inclusion of environmental measures and the engagement of diverse communities in genomics research. Funding agencies and research institutions should develop strategies to encourage and reward such collaborations.

The recommendations in this report have been developed from the committee's collective experience researching, writing about, and using population descriptors. But there is more that can be done to understand how population descriptors are used in genetics and genomics research and the effects that these descriptors have in medicine and in health disparities studies.

Recommendation 11. Given the persistent need to address this dynamic, high-stakes component of genomics research, funders and research institutions should create new initiatives to advance the study and methods development of best practices for population descriptor usage in genetics and genomics research, including the public availability of resources.

Recommendation 12. Key partners, including funding agencies, research institutions, and scientific journals, should ensure that policies and procedures are aligned with these recommendations and invest in developing new strategies to support implementation when needed.

MECHANISMS OF ACCOUNTABILITY

The ability of this report to effect durable change rests on three principles: actionable recommendations, implementation procedures applied effectively across the genomics ecosystem, and, importantly, accountability mechanisms. Accountability serves multiple purposes. First, the committee recognizes that the usefulness of today's population descriptors in research will not necessarily be valid in the future. Thus, there will be a need for a body to periodically evaluate current population descriptors and recommend changes based on both sociological and scientific data and ethical and empirical principles. In addition, this or a second oversight body needs sufficient powers to monitor and facilitate the implementation of the report's recommendations. For example, this group could monitor what journals are doing; convene journal editors and publishers to formulate consistent, reasonable guidelines; and help them standardize their instructions to authors, so researchers recognize that all of the journals are following identical standards. This body could perform similar facilitative functions for funding agencies, and assist agencies, research institutions, and professional societies in developing training as well as ways to measure the effectiveness of the training over time. To be respected, trusted, and effective, it would be best for this body (or these bodies) to comprise people from all of the relevant parties within the genetics and genomics ecosystem. Perhaps the National Institutes of Health's Advisory Committee on Research on Women's Health or the Novel and Exceptional Technology and Research Advisory Committee[15] could serve as examples on which such a body could be modeled.

> **Recommendation 13. Because the understanding of population descriptors in genomics research is continuously evolving, responsibility for periodic reevaluation of these recommendations should be overseen by effective, multidisciplinary advisory groups. Such advisory groups could:**
> - periodically reevaluate established best practices on the use of descent-associated population descriptors to ensure they reflect the current state of the science and ongoing commitment to ethical and empirical principles;
> - advise funders and other relevant parties on the use of population descriptors and their implementation;
> - facilitate the coordination of international best practice sharing;
> - provide a venue for input from the broader community, including research participants; and
> - monitor and measure changes adopted by funders, researchers, journals, societies, and other relevant parties based on the uptake of best practices identified.

PARTING THOUGHTS

Despite the many recommendations, guidelines, and strategies promoting the ethically and empirically sound use of descent-associated population descriptors, there has been relatively little change in how any entities within the genetics and genomics research ecosystem use these descriptors or require them to be used. It will take a concerted and interdisciplinary effort by all interested parties, patience, and a good bit of time to reach a place where the proper use and reporting of population descriptors is routine. Individual researchers will bear the brunt of these changes, so it will be essential for their institutions and funders, along with journal editors and professional societies, to form a supportive and adequately resourced network that makes this transition feasible. The recommendations in this report will need to be implemented broadly and consistently, by all of the relevant parties,

---

[15] https://orwh.od.nih.gov/about/advisory-committees/advisory-committee-on-research-on-womens-health (accessed January 3, 2023).

to generate lasting change. The committee hopes that by having identified the roles that each party plays and by developing mechanisms that facilitate transparency and good communication among all interested parties, the scale of the tasks will be manageable to meet the needs of this evolving field.

REFERENCES

AAA (American Anthropological Association). 1997. *American Anthropological Association response to OMB Directive 15: Race and ethnic standards for federal statistics and administrative reporting.* https://s3.amazonaws.com/rdcms-aaa/files/production/public/FileDownloads/pdfs/cmtes/minority/upload/AAA_Response_OMB1997.pdf (accessed August 31, 2022).

AAA. 1998. *AAA statement on race.* https://www.americananthro.org/ConnectWithAAA/Content.aspx?ItemNumber=2583 (accessed December 6, 2022).

AAPA (American Association of Physical Anthropology). 1996. AAPA statement on biological aspects of race. *American Association of Physical Anthropology* 101:569-570.

All of Us. 2022. *Register to be an All of Us researcher.* https://www.researchallofus.org/register/ (accessed December 6, 2022).

AMA (American Medical Association). 2020a. *Elimination of race as a proxy for ancestry, genetics, and biology in medical education, research and clinical practice.* Chicago, IL: American Medical Association.

AMA. 2020b. *New AMA policies recognize race as a social, not biological, construct.* Chicago, IL: American Medical Association.

APA (American Psychological Association). 2003. Guidelines on multicultural education, training, research, practice, and organizational change for psychologists. *American Psychology* 58(5):377-402.

APA. 2017. *Multicultural guidelines: An ecological approach to context, identity, and intersectionality, 2017.* https://www.apa.org/about/policy/multicultural-guidelines.pdf (accessed December 6, 2022).

APA, APA Task Force on Race and Ethnicity Guidelines in Psychology. 2019. *APA guidelines on race and ethnicity in psychology: Promoting responsiveness and equity.* https://www.apa.org/about/policy/guidelines-race-ethnicity.pdf (accessed December 6, 2022).

APA. 2022. *EDI efforts: Journal equity, diversity, and inclusion statement.* https://www.apa.org/pubs/journals/amp?tab=6#tabs (accessed December 6, 2022).

Bailey, Z. D., J. M. Feldman, and M. T. Bassett. 2020. How structural racism works—racist policies as a root cause of U.S. racial health inequities. *New England Journal of Medicine* 384(8):768-773.

Borrell, L. N., J. R. Elhawary, E. Fuentes-Afflick, J. Witonsky, N. Bhakta, A. H. B. Wu, K. Bibbins-Domingo, J. R. Rodríguez-Santana, M. A. Lenoir, J. R. Gavin, III, R. A. Kittles, N. A. Zaitlen, D. S. Wilkes, N. R. Powe, E. Ziv, and E. G. Burchard. 2021. Race and genetic ancestry in medicine—A time for reckoning with racism. *New England Journal of Medicine* 384(5):474-480.

Churchwell, K., M. S. V. Elkind, R. M. Benjamin, A. P. Carson, E. K. Chang, W. Lawrence, A. Mills, T. M. Odom, C. J. Rodriguez, F. Rodriguez, E. Sanchez, A. Z. Sharrief, M. Sims, and O. Williams. 2020. Call to action: Structural racism as a fundamental driver of health disparities: A presidential advisory from the American Heart Association. *Circulation* 142(24):e454-e468.

CTSA (Clinical Translational Science Awards) Consortium, and Community Engagement Key Function Committee Task Force on the Principles of Community Engagement. 2011. *Principles of community engagement (2nd edition)*. Department of Health and Human Services.

Flanagin, A., T. Frey, and S. L. Christiansen. 2021. Updated guidance on the reporting of race and ethnicity in medical and science journals. *JAMA* 326(7):621.

Fuentes, A., R. R. Ackermann, S. Athreya, D. Bolnick, T. Lasisi, S. H. Lee, S. A. McLean, and R. Nelson. 2019. AAPA statement on race and racism. *American Journal of Physical Anthropology* 169(3):400-402.

Hunt, L. M., and M. S. Megyesi. 2008. The ambiguous meanings of the racial/ethnic categories routinely used in human genetics research. *Social Science and Medicine* 66(2):349-361.

IOM (Institute of Medicine). 2009. *Race, ethnicity, and language data: Standardization for health care quality improvement*. Edited by C. Ulmer, B. McFadden, and D. R. Nerenz. Washington, DC: The National Academies Press.

Kaplan, J. B., and T. Bennett. 2003. Use of race and ethnicity in biomedical publication. *JAMA* 289(20):2709-2716.

Roman, Y. 2022. The United States 2020 census data: Implications for precision medicine and the research landscape. *Personalized Medicine* 19(1).

Takezawa, Y., K. Kato, H. Oota, T. Caulfield, A. Fujimoto, S. Honda, N. Kamatani, S. Kawamura, K. Kawashima, R. Kimura, H. Matsumae, A. Saito, P. E. Savage, N. Seguchi, K. Shimizu, S. Terao, Y. Yamaguchi-Kabata, A. Yasukouchi, M. Yoneda, and K. Tokunaga. 2014. Human genetics research, race, ethnicity and the labeling of populations: Recommendations based on an interdisciplinary workshop in Japan. *BMC Medical Ethics* 15(1).

A

Study Approach and Methods

The committee was asked to produce a report that identifies best practices on the use of race, ethnicity, genetic ancestry, and other population descriptors in genetics and genomics research. To respond to this charge, the committee drew upon the expertise of its members and reviewed data from many sources using targeted outreach to relevant parties, the existing literature, and public input gathered via a series of public meetings and workshops.

EXPERTISE

The committee was composed of 17 members with expertise in diverse areas including human genetics, population genetics, clinical genetics, genetic epidemiology, statistical and computational genetics and genomics, anthropology, sociology, social epidemiology, demography and population statistics, and historical, ethical, legal, and social implications research. Committee biographies can be found in Appendix E.

OUTREACH

The committee was especially interested in obtaining input from researchers, advocates, publishers, and other interested public parties on the effectiveness of current population descriptors in genomics research and the future use of population descriptors. To that end, the committee issued a call for public comments on March 9, 2022, that was open until June 1, 2022. The announcement was shared on the study webpage, shared as an email sent to Health and Medicine Division (HMD) listservs, and posted on various social media platforms. The request focused on comments related to a series of questions:

- How do you identify yourself, and how do you think that should be incorporated into genetics research studies?
- How are population descriptors such as race, ethnicity, and ancestry being used or not used effectively in genomics research?
- What population descriptors, if any, should not be used in genomics research?
- Do all genetics studies need specific population and/or individual descriptors of their study participants?
- What aspects of the current use of population descriptors in genomics research need to be changed or improved?
- How should population descriptors be used in genomics research moving forward?

Comments received from the public were shared with the committee and included in the committee's public access file. Several members of the public who submitted public comments were invited to share their remarks during public comment sessions at the committee's virtual public workshops.

LITERATURE REVIEW

Literature relevant to the committee's charge was identified from multiple sources, including targeted staff searches and reviews of previous efforts to identify best practices for the use of population descriptors. National Academies staff conducted a literature search using the databases Embase, Medline, and Scopus. These databases index research in biomedicine, health sciences, and other fields; they were searched January 17–20, 2022. Search terms, including MeSH terms,[1] comprised vocabulary related to categorization and labeling, disparities, concepts of race, and genetics (see Table A-1). Publications in English were included across all demographics and global locations. The timeframe of publication was limited to 1990 to date. Committee members, speakers, and members of the public also submitted relevant articles and comments on the committee's charge.

---

[1] MeSH terms are from the Medical Subject Headings thesaurus used to index research in the life sciences and enable use of a hierarchical search structure.

TABLE A-1 Literature Search Terms

Group A	Group B	Group C	Group D
Categories	Bias, implicit/	Ancestry	Biotechnology/
Categorization	Bias/	Concepts of	Genetics,
Classification	Discrimination	race	population/
Controlled vocabulary	Disparities	Constructs of	Genetics/
Data collection/	Diversity	race	Genetic testing/
Databases, genetic/	Equity	Demography/	Genome, human/
Databases as topic/	Health inequities/	Ethnic groups/	Genomics/
Datasets	Health status	Ethnicity/	Genotype
Datasets as topic/	disparities/	Ethnogenetic	Human genetics/
Descriptors	Implicit bias	Ethnoracial	Human genome
Forms as topic/	Inequalities	Heredity	Pharmacogenetics/
Keywords	Inequity	Population	Pharmacogenomics
Labeling	Nondiscrimination	demographics	Population genetics
Medical records/	Prejudice/	Population	
Metadata/	Racism/	groups/	
Nomenclature	Stereotyping/	Race	
OMB descriptors	Systemic racism/	Racial groups/	
Office of Management and			
Budget			
Questionnaires			
Race categories			
Racial categories			
Race variables			
Racial variables			
Race models			
Registers			
Registry			
Reporting			
Screening			
Self-report/			
Subject headings/			
Surveys			
Surveys and questionnaires/			
Systematized Nomenclature of			
Medicine/			
Terminology			
Terminology as topic/			
Vocabulary			
Vocabulary, controlled/			

NOTE: / indicates MeSH terms. The search strategy consisted of Group A + Group B + Group C + Group D.
SOURCE: National Academies staff, January 20, 2022.

PUBLIC MEETINGS

The committee convened three public meetings and gathered information from invited expert speakers and members of the public. The committee's first meeting was held virtually in February 2022, and the public session provided an opportunity for the committee to clarify questions related to the statement of task with the sponsoring organization. Subsequent public workshops were held virtually on April 4, 2022, and June 14, 2022. The agendas for these meetings are included in chronological order.

First Committee Meeting, Open Session

February 14, 2022

Session Objective: To hear from the sponsors of the study regarding their perspectives on the charge to the committee.

12:30 p.m. ET	**Welcome and Goals for the Session** ARAVINDA CHAKRAVARTI, New York University, Committee Co-Chair CHARMAINE ROYAL, Duke University, Committee Co-Chair
12:40 p.m.	**NIH Presents the Charge to the Committee** Presenter: ERIC GREEN, Director, National Human Genome Research Institute Panelists: • VENCE BONHAM, Acting Deputy Director, National Human Genome Research Institute • STEPHEN CHANOCK, Director, Division of Cancer Epidemiology & Genetics, National Cancer Institute • ELISEO J. PÉREZ-STABLE, Director, National Institute on Minority Health and Health Disparities • SHERI SCHULLY, Deputy Chief Medical and Scientific Officer, *All of Us* Research Program
1:10 p.m.	**Discussion and Q&A with Committee**
2:00 p.m.	**Adjourn Day 1**

Public Workshop

April 4, 2022

11:00 a.m. ET   **Welcome and Goals for the Workshop**
ARAVINDA CHAKRAVARTI, *Committee Cochair*
Director, Center for Human Genetics and Genomics
Muriel G. & George W. Singer Professor of
     Neuroscience & Physiology
New York University Grossman School of Medicine

CHARMAINE ROYAL, *Committee Cochair*
Robert O. Keohane Professor of African & African
     American Studies, Biology, Global Health, and
     Family Medicine & Community Health
Director, Duke Center on Genomics, Race, Identity,
     Difference and Duke Center for Truth, Racial
     Healing & Transformation
Duke University

Session I: Historical and Current Use of Population Descriptors in
Genomics Research
Moderator: Sandra Soo-Jin Lee, Columbia University

Session Objectives:
- To explore historical use of population descriptors to better understand current use
- To examine whom researchers study in genomics investigations
- To explore why researchers identify individuals and populations in genomics studies
- To examine and identify the criticisms and challenges in current use of population descriptors in genomics research

11:10 a.m.   **Brief Introduction to the Session by the Moderator**

11:15 a.m.   **Speakers' Talks (15 minutes each)**
PILAR OSSORIO
Professor of Law and Bioethics
University of Wisconsin-Madison, Law School
University of Wisconsin-Madison, Medical School

Joseph Graves, Jr.
Professor of Biological Sciences
PI: IBIEM@AT and BEACON@A&T
Associate Director, Triangle Center for Evolutionary
    Medicine
Department of Biology
North Carolina A&T State University

Andrew Clark
Jacob Gould Schurman Professor of Population
    Genetics
Nancy and Peter Meinin Family Investigator
Associate Director, Cornell Center for Comparative
    and Population Genomics
Interim Chair, Department of Computational Biology
Cornell University

Rina Bliss
Associate Professor of Sociology
Rutgers University

12:15 p.m.   **Q&A with Speakers**

1:00 p.m.   **Break**

Session II: Future Use of Population Descriptors in Genomics Research
Moderator: Rick Kittles, City of Hope

Session Objectives:
- To consider the diverse types of population and individual de-
  scriptors (e.g., origins, definitions, and usage in the United States,
  implications for non-U.S. participants)
- To discuss possible ideal descriptors of populations and individuals
- To consider standardized or ideal systems of population descriptors

1:30 p.m.   **Brief Introduction to the Session by the Moderator**

1:35 p.m.   **Speakers' Talks (15 minutes each)**

Tesfaye Mersha
Associate Professor of Human Quantitative Genetics
Department of Pediatrics
University of Cincinnati
Cincinnati Children's Hospital Medical Center

MELINDA MILLS
Director, Leverhulme Centre for Demographic Sciences
Nuffield Professor of Sociology
University of Oxford

JOANNA MOUNTAIN
Consultant
23andMe

EIMEAR KENNY
Founding Director, Institute for Genomic Health
Professor of Genetics and Medicine
Icahn School of Medicine at Mount Sinai

STEPHANIE MALIA FULLERTON
Professor of Bioethics and Humanities
University of Washington School of Medicine
Adjunct Professor
Departments of Epidemiology, Genome Sciences,
     and Medicine
University of Washington
Affiliate Investigator, Public Health Sciences Division
Fred Hutchinson Cancer Research Center

2:55 p.m.   **Q&A with Speakers**

3:50 p.m.   **Break**

Session III: Community Input on Population Descriptors in Genomics
Research
*Moderator: Katrina Claw, University of Colorado Denver – Anschutz
Medical Campus*

Session Objectives:
- To hear from a variety of interested parties on the following topics:
    - What works and does not work about the current population
      descriptors used in genomics research?
    - What could be improved in current use of population descrip-
      tors in genomics research?

4:00 p.m.   **Brief Introduction to the Session by the Moderator**

4:05 p.m.   **Speakers' Comments (5 minutes each)**

CATHERINE POTENSKI
Chief Editor
Nature Genetics

DONNA CRYER
President and CEO
Global Liver Institute

AGUSTÍN FUENTES
Professor
Department of Anthropology
Princeton University

CHARLES ROTIMI
President
American Society for Human Genetics

JUDIT KUMUTHINI
Bioinformatics Manager
Human Capacity Development Manager:
Bioinformatics
University of Western Cape

SHISHI LUO
Associate Director, Bioinformatics and Infectious
    Diseases
Helix Genomics

JULIA ORTEGA
Vice President
iHope Genetic Health
Genetic Alliance

KEOLU FOX
Assistant Professor
Department of Anthropology
University of California, San Diego

4:55 p.m.   **Concluding Remarks**

5:00 p.m.   **Adjourn**

Public Workshop

June 14, 2022

12:30–12:40 p.m. ET   **Welcome and Goals for the Workshop**
CHARMAINE ROYAL, *Committee Cochair*
Robert O. Keohane Professor of African &
      African American Studies, Biology, Global
      Health, and Family Medicine &
      Community Health
Director, Duke Center on Genomics, Race,
      Identity, Difference and Duke Center
      for Truth, Racial Healing & Transformation
Duke University

ARAVINDA CHAKRAVARTI, *Committee Cochair*
Director, Center for Human Genetics and
      Genomics
Muriel G. & George W. Singer Professor of
      Neuroscience & Physiology
New York University Grossman School
      of Medicine

Session I: Examining Use of Population Descriptors in Genomics Research
Moderator: John Novembre, University of Chicago

Session Objectives:
- To explore what types of population descriptors are needed for genetics and genomics studies
- What is a genetics study trying to accomplish?
- Who is sampled? Why are they sampled? What are participants called, and why?
- To examine how and why genetics studies should or should not incorporate social categories and environmental factors

12:40–12:45 p.m.   **Brief Introduction to the Session**

JOHN NOVEMBRE
Professor, Department of Human Genetics,
      Department of Ecology & Evolution
University of Chicago

12:45–1:45 p.m.	**Speakers' Talks**

GIL MCVEAN
Professor of Statistical Genetics
Director, Big Data Institute
Fellow of Linacre College
University of Oxford

AKINYEMI ONI-ORISAN
Assistant Professor, Department of Clinical
  Pharmacy
University of California, San Francisco School of
  Pharmacy

NANCY COX
Director, Vanderbilt Genetics Institute
Director, Division of Genetic Medicine
Mary Phillips Edmonds Gray Professor of
  Genetics
Vanderbilt University

GRAHAM COOP
Professor, Department of Evolution and Ecology
  and Center for Population Biology
University of California, Davis

1:45–2:25 p.m.	**Q&A with Speakers**
2:25–2:40 p.m.	**Break**

Session II: Use of Population Descriptors by Biobanks and Other
Research Consortia
Moderator: Ann Morning, New York University

Session Objectives:
- To examine how and why biobanks use taxonomies currently, es-
  pecially in areas of large diversity
- To explore how legacy data might be managed and merged with
  future data
- To learn how large-scale data collection projects are designed

2:40–2:45 p.m.	**Brief Introduction to the Session**
	ANN MORNING
	Associate Professor, Department of Sociology
	Academic Director, 19 Washington Square North
	(NYU Abu Dhabi in NY)
	New York University

2:45–3:30 p.m.   **Speakers' Talks**

PHIL TSAO
Professor (Research), Medicine – Cardiovascular
    Medicine
Stanford University

ALICE POPEJOY
Assistant Professor, Department of Public Health
    Sciences
University of California, Davis

MASHAAL SOHAIL
Associate Professor, Center for Genomic Sciences
National Autonomous University of Mexico

3:30–4:00 p.m.   **Q&A with Speakers**

4:00–4:10 p.m.   **Break**

Session III: Community Input on Population Descriptors in Genomics
Research
Moderator: Charmaine Royal, Duke University

Session Objective:
- To hear from a variety of interested parties on the following topics:
  - What works and does not work about the current population
    descriptors used in genomics research?
  - What could be improved in the current use of population de-
    scriptors in genomics research?

4:10–4:15 p.m.   **Introduction to the Session**
CHARMAINE ROYAL
Robert O. Keohane Professor of African &
    African American Studies, Biology, Global
    Health, and Family Medicine & Community
    Health
Director, Duke Center on Genomics, Race,
    Identity, Difference and Duke Center for
    Truth, Racial Healing & Transformation
Duke University

4:15–4:55 p.m.   **Speakers' Comments**

JENNIFER WEBSTER
Senior Director, Precision Medicine RWE Lead
Pfizer

SANTIAGO MOLINA
Postdoctoral Fellow, Sociology/Science in Human
    Culture
Department of Sociology
Weinberg College of Arts & Sciences
Northwestern University

NORBERT TAVARES
Program Manager, Cell Biology
Chan-Zuckerberg Initiative

KING JORDAN
Professor, School of Biological Sciences
Director, Bioinformatics Graduate Program
Georgia Institute of Technology

DIANALEE McKNIGHT
Medical Affairs Director, Emerging Clinical
    Omics
Invitae

RAMYA M. RAJAGOPALAN
Associate Director, Training, Evaluation, and
    Qualitative Research
Center for Empathy and Technology, T. Denny
    Sanford Institute for Empathy and
    Compassion
University of California, San Diego

STACY CHRISTIANSEN
Managing Editor, *JAMA*
Chair, AMA Manual of Styles

HANNAH WAND
Director, Preventive Genomics Program
Genetics Counselor
Stanford Health Care

4:55–5:00 p.m.   **Concluding Remarks**

5:00 p.m.   **Adjourn**

B

Glossary

Admixture: An individual is described as *admixed* when they have lines of ancestry that trace back to multiple distant geographic origins on a recent timescale: as an example, individuals of Central and South America whose ancestry 600 years ago traces to individuals mostly living in western Europe, west Africa, and Central/South America (Winkler et al., 2010). A difficulty with the concept is the often-implicit timescale being considered. All humans are admixed, but not everyone is recently admixed: for some, ancestry lines will trace back to geographically distant ancestors within a few generations, whereas for others, the same process occurs on much longer timescales. A further challenge is the framing of admixture as the blending of "source populations," which may erroneously imply the existence of homogeneous populations in the past.

Ancestral recombination graph: For a set of individuals, the graph depicting the genetic ancestry lines (or paths) that trace back to their common genetic ancestors at every position in the genome (Hudson, 1990).

Ancestry: a person's origin or descent, lineage, "roots," or heritage, including kinship (U.S. Census, 2021). Commonly associated with genealogical ancestry—that is, the collection of ancestors for an individual as found in a family tree, including parents, grandparents, great-grandparents, and so on (Mathieson and Scally, 2020). Examples of ancestry group labels include clan names or patronyms, but geographic, ethnicity, or racial labels are often used to denote groups whose members are presumed to share common ancestry. See also *Genealogical ancestors, Genetic ancestors, Genetic ancestry, Genetic ancestry group,* and *Genetic similarity.*

Ancient DNA: DNA extracted from individuals who died anywhere from tens to many thousands of years ago (ISOGG, 2020). Studies using ancient DNA often integrate genetic data with archeological and historical data to make inferences about modern population origins.

Continental groupings: labels based on the continent of origin of an individual. These groupings do not account for the substantial genetic, environmental, and geographic diversity within continents (Lewis et al., 2022). For example, in the United States, both someone from Japan and someone from India are often labeled as Asian.

Culture: the dimension of human life including behavior, objects, and ideas that appear to express, or to stand for, something else. These include values, norms, beliefs, symbols, and symbolically meaningful practices like foodways or religious worship (Griswold, 2013).

Environment: the complex of physical, social, cultural, chemical, and biotic factors that act upon a person (Merriam-Webster, n.d.). Environment can also refer to a person's exposure to chemicals and toxins, biological exposures, diet, behavioral patterns, life events, or even to more macroenvironmental exposures such as neighborhood air pollution and violence (Glass and McAtee, 2006; Ottman, 1996).

Epidemiology: the study of the distribution and determinants of risk factors of disease, how these factors determine the incidence and prevalence of disease in human populations, and the application of this research to control health problems (Aschengrau and Seage, 2020).

Epigenetics: the science that studies alterations in gene function through chromatin modifications and chemical changes to an individual's DNA that do not involve alterations of the underlying nucleotide sequence (Cazaly et al., 2019; Hurle, 2022).

Ethnicity: a sociopolitically constructed system for classifying human beings according to claims of shared heritage often based on perceived cultural similarities (e.g., language, religion, beliefs); the system varies globally. In the United States, ethnic group labels often derive from the country of origin for voluntary immigrants (e.g., Italian Americans, Korean Americans). Outside the United States, ethnicity can denote groups that are considered indigenous to a given territory; therefore, globally, ethnicity is not limited to a product of migration.

Evolution: change in allele frequencies or heritable traits over successive generations, which arises from the interplay of mutation, recombination, migration, genetic drift, and natural selection (Emlen and Zimmer, 2020).

Genealogical ancestors: the set of biological ancestors in an individual's family tree or pedigree, including parents, grandparents, great-grandparents, etc. Not all of an individual's genealogical ancestors are their genetic ancestors, that is, have contributed DNA to that focal individual (Mathieson and Scally, 2020); in fact, most did not (Coop, 2017). See also *Ancestry, Genetic ancestors, Genetic ancestry, Genetic ancestry group*, and *Genetic similarity*.

Genetic ancestors: the subset of genealogical ancestors who transmitted DNA to a focal individual (Donnelly, 1983). See also *Ancestry, Genealogical ancestors, Genetic ancestry, Genetic ancestry group*, and *Genetic similarity*.

Genetic ancestry: the paths through an individual's family tree by which they have inherited DNA from specific ancestors (Mathieson and Scally, 2020). Genetic ancestry can be thought of in terms of lines extending upwards in a family tree from an individual through their genetic ancestors (see Figure 2-1). Shared genetic ancestry arises from having genetic ancestors in common (that is, overlapping lines of ancestry). For a set of individuals, a fundamental representation of genetic ancestry is a structure called an ancestral recombination graph (Mathieson and Scally, 2020). In practice, shared genetic ancestry is typically inferred by some measure(s) of genetic similarity. See also *Ancestral recombination graph, Ancestry, Genealogical ancestors, Genetic ancestors, Genetic ancestry group*, and *Genetic similarity*.

Genetic ancestry group: a set of individuals who share more similar genetic ancestries. In practice, a genetic ancestry group is constituted based on some measure(s) of genetic similarity (Coop, 2022; Mathieson and Scally, 2020). Once a set is designated as a genetic ancestry group, its members are often assigned a geographic, ethnic, or other nongenetic label that is common among its members. See also *Ancestry, Genealogical ancestors, Genetic ancestors, Genetic ancestry*, and *Genetic similarity*.

Genetic epidemiology: the study of the role of genes and environmental factors, and their interactions, as risk factors in the occurrence of disease and traits in populations (Duggal et al., 2019; Seyerle and Avery, 2013).

Genetic similarity: quantitative measure of the genetic resemblance between individuals that reflects the extent of shared genetic ancestry (e.g., the mean number of genotype differences between individuals) (Mathieson and Scally, 2020). See also *Ancestry, Genealogical ancestors, Genetic ancestors, Genetic ancestry,* and *Genetic ancestry group.*

Genetics: the science of heredity, specifically the mechanisms by which traits or characteristics (phenotypes) are transmitted from one generation to the next as well as how genes influence phenotypes (King et al., 2014).

Genome: the totality of an individual's DNA in all chromosomes, including the mitochondria, comprising all genes, their regulatory machinery, and genomic architectural elements (Green, 2022a).

Genome-wide association study (GWAS): a method to associate variation in trait values (e.g., disease risk or height) with specific genetic variants in the genome (Hutter, 2022). Only a subset of associated variants is expected to be causal for the trait, as many genetic variants will only be associated owing to their correlation with the causal variants (e.g., due to linkage disequilibrium) (Hirschhorn and Daly, 2005).

Genomics: the science and technologies of studying the structure and function of the entire genome (Green, 2022b).

Group label: name given to a population that describes or classifies it according to the dimension along which it was identified. An example is *French* as the label for a group identified by its members' possession of French nationality, where *nationality* is the population descriptor. See also *Population descriptor.*

Hierarchical thinking: a process of ranking people or things in regard to status; in the context of this study, this thinking assumes that one group of people is superior to another.

Human genetics: the science of genes, chromosomes, and the information they encode in human heredity.

Identity-by-descent: segments of the genome inherited by two or more people from the same relatively recent ancestor are referred to as identical-by-descent; such segments are often identified based on their high genetic similarity (or "identity-by-state") (Thompson, 2013).

Indigeneity: a population classification or descriptor that, like ethnicity, carries connotations of descent-associated cultural traditions. Indigeneity is distinguished from other population descriptors, however, by its emphasis on the continuity of geographic location over time. Indigenous people are the aboriginal inhabitants of a land in contrast to later migrant or colonizer populations; there are many histories of colonization resulting in dislocation of Indigenous peoples from their lands and interruption of traditional lifestyles and culture (Mudd-Martin et al., 2021).

Labeling scheme: a framework for assigning labels to human participants in a study.

Natural selection: the process whereby some individuals, better adapted to their surroundings, are more likely to survive and leave descendants. If a trait under selection is heritable, natural selection can lead to change in trait values over generations through changes in causal allele frequencies (Emlen and Zimmer, 2020).

Phenotype: an observable trait of an individual, which arises from genetic and environmental effects and often their interaction (NHGRI, 2022; Shriner, 2013).

Polygenic score (PGS): a score (also called polygenic risk score or polygenic index) for an individual based on a set of variants associated with a trait (Manolio, 2022). In practice, this is done by summing the alleles the person carries at these causal factors, weighted by the effect sizes on the trait (estimated in a prior GWAS) (Sirugo et al., 2019). A PGS provides a predictor of the deviation from a mean value in a given study population. The hope is to use PGS to identify individuals at risk for specific diseases or to disentangle genetic and environmental effects on a trait (Kullo et al., 2022).

Population: a group of humans that is identified by a selected dimension or characteristic (or set of dimensions or characteristics) for the purposes of analysis; this definition does *not* assume that all the group's members are identical or homogenous. For example, college students in the United States represent an identifiable population. In statistics, the concept of a population is foundational and represents a set of individuals or objects with shared identifying characteristics that is studied indirectly through observations of random samples. In population genetic theory, the concept of a population is often defined as a group with a common gene pool from which individuals choose mates with whom they reproduce (King et al., 2014), often assumed not to experience immigration or emigration (e.g., in some models, a population is characterized by a set of allele frequencies). In population genetic analysis, the concept is much like the definition in statistics.

Population descriptor: a concept or classification scheme that categorizes people into groups (or "populations") according to a perceived characteristic or dimension of interest. A few examples include race, ethnicity, and geographic location, although this is a non-exhaustive list. The salience of a given population descriptor may vary from place to place, so descriptors (and/or their associated group labels) that are used in the United States may not be widespread in other countries. See also *Group label* and *Labeling scheme*.

Race: a sociopolitically constructed system for classifying and ranking human beings according to subjective beliefs about shared ancestry based on perceived innate biological similarities; the system varies globally. Race is founded on the belief that there are naturally and innately distinct groups that can be identified. This perspective has been used to justify the unequal distribution of resources from land and labor to power and status. In short, race is the product of racism rather than the other way around. As a social construct or a social invention with political, economic, and historical context (ASA, 2003; Morning, 2005), race is both an idea and a way of organizing society that varies over time and from place to place.

Taxonomy: a system of classification. The explicit or implicit schema used to define categories and labels for a set of individuals (or populations) constitutes a taxonomy.

Typological thinking: a way of classifying individuals in terms of set types to which they belong while disregarding variation among individuals within the type; often reinforces long-standing prejudice about characteristics of groups (Lewens, 2009).

REFERENCES

ASA (American Sociological Association). 2003. *The importance of collecting data and doing social scientific research on race.* Washington, DC: American Sociological Association.

Aschengrau, A., and G. R. Seage III. 2020. *Essentials of epidemiology in public health.* 4th ed. Burlington, MA: Jones & Bartlett Learning.

Cazaly, E., J. Saad, W. Wang, C. Heckman, M. Ollikainen, and J. Tang. 2019. Making sense of the epigenome using data integration approaches. *Frontiers in Pharmacology* 10.

Coop, G. 2017. *Our vast, shared family tree.* https://gcbias.org/2017/11/20/our-vast-shared-family-tree/ (accessed November 7, 2022).

Coop, G. 2023. Genetic similarity versus genetic ancestry groups as sample descriptors in human genetics. *arXiv* (pre-print).

Donnelly, K. P. 1983. The probability that related individuals share some section of genome identical by descent. *Theoretical Population Biology* 23(1):34-63.

Duggal, P., C. Ladd-Acosta, D. Ray, and T. H. Beaty. 2019. The evolving field of genetic epidemiology: From familial aggregation to genomic sequencing. *American Journal of Epidemiology* 188(12):2069-2077.

Emlen, D. J., and C. Zimmer. 2020. *Evolution: Making sense of life.* 3rd ed. New York: Macmillian Learning.

Glass, T. A., and M. J. McAtee. 2006. Behavioral science at the crossroads in public health: Extending horizons, envisioning the future. *Social Science & Medicine* 62(7):1650-1671.

Green, E. 2022a. *Genome.* https://www.genome.gov/genetics-glossary/Genome (accessed November 11, 2022).

Green, E. 2022b. *Genomics.* https://www.genome.gov/genetics-glossary/genomics (accessed November 11, 2022).

Griswold, W. 2013. *Cultures and societies in a changing world.* 4th ed. Thousand Oaks, CA: SAGE.

Hirschhorn, J. N., and M. J. Daly. 2005. Genome-wide association studies for common diseases and complex traits. *Nature Reviews Genetics* 6(2):95-108.

Hudson, R. R. 1990. Gene genealogies and the coalescent process. *Oxford Surveys in Evolutionary Biology* 7(1):44.

Hurle, B. 2022. *Epigenetics.* https://www.genome.gov/genetics-glossary/Epigenetics (accessed October 19, 2022).

Hutter, C. M. 2022. *Genome-wide association studies (GWAS).* https://www.genome.gov/genetics-glossary/Genome-Wide-Association-Studies?id=91 (accessed October 19, 2022).

ISOGG (International Society of Genetic Genealogy). 2020. *Ancient DNA.* https://isogg.org/wiki/Ancient_DNA (accessed November 11, 2022).

King, R. C., P. K. Mulligan, and W. D. Stansfield. 2014. *A dictionary of genetics.* 8th ed. Oxford University Press.

Kullo, I. J., C. M. Lewis, M. Inouye, A. R. Martin, S. Ripatti, and N. Chatterjee. 2022. Polygenic scores in biomedical research. *Nature Reviews Genetics* 23(9):524-532.

Lewens, T. 2009. What is wrong with typological thinking? *Philosophy of Science* 76(3): 355-371.

Lewis, A. C. F., S. J. Molina, P. S. Appelbaum, B. Dauda, A. Di Rienzo, A. Fuentes, S. M. Fullerton, N. A. Garrison, N. Ghosh, E. M. Hammonds, D. S. Jones, E. E. Kenny, P. Kraft, S. S. Lee, M. Mauro, J. Novembre, A. Panofsky, M. Sohail, B. M. Neale, and D. S. Allen. 2022. Getting genetic ancestry right for science and society. *Science* 376(6590):250-252.

Manolio, T. 2022. *Polygenic risk score (PRS).* https://www.genome.gov/genetics-glossary/Polygenic-Risk-Score (accessed November 11, 2022).

Mathieson, I., and A. Scally. 2020. What is ancestry? *PLoS Genetics* 16(3):e1008624.

Merriam-Webster. n.d. Environment. In *Merriam-Webster.com dictionary.* https://www.merriam-webster.com/dictionary/environment (accessed December 7, 2022).

Morning, A. 2005. Keyword: Race. *Contexts* 4(4):44-46.

Mudd-Martin, G., A. L. Cirino, V. Barcelona, K. Fox, M. Hudson, Y. V. Sun, J. Y. Taylor, and V. A. Cameron. 2021. Considerations for cardiovascular genetic and genomic research with marginalized racial and ethnic groups and Indigenous peoples: A scientific statement from the American Heart Association. *Circulation: Genomic and Precision Medicine* 14(4):e000084.

NHGRI (National Human Genome Research Institute). 2022. *Evolution.* https://www.genome.gov/genetics-glossary/Evolution (accessed December 6, 2022).

Ottman, R. 1996. Gene–environment interaction: Definitions and study designs. *Preventive Medicine* 25(6):764-770.

Seyerle, A. A., and C. L. Avery. 2013. Genetic epidemiology: The potential benefits and challenges of using genetic information to improve human health. *North Carolina Medical Journal* 74(6):505-508.

Shriner, D. 2013. Overview of admixture mapping. *Current Protocols in Human Genetics* 94:1-23.

Sirugo, G., S. M. Williams, and S. A. Tishkoff. 2019. The missing diversity in human genetic studies. *Cell* 177(1):26-31.

Thompson, E. A. 2013. Identity by descent: Variation in meiosis, across genomes, and in populations. *Genetics* 194(2):301-326.

U.S. Census. 2021. *About ancestry.* https://www.census.gov/topics/population/ancestry/about. html#:~:text=Ancestry%20refers%20to%20a%20person's,arrival%20in%20the%20 United%20States (accessed November 11, 2022).

Winkler, C. A., G. W. Nelson, and M. W. Smith. 2010. Admixture mapping comes of age. *Annual Review of Genomics and Human Genetics* 11(1):65-89.

C

Table of International Programs

TABLE C-1 International Programs

Name	Country/Region	Short Description	Population Descriptors Used
BioBank Japan (BBJ)	Japan	BBJ was started in 2003 as a disease biobank. Since 2018, the aim of the biobank is to use the registered samples and data for genomics and clinical research (BBJ, 2021).	None
Brazilian Initiative on Precision Medicine (BIPMed)	Brazil	The aim is to offer public access to genomic and phenotypic data from Brazil to scientists and clinicians around the world. It is the Brazilian Country Node of the Human Variome Project (HVP) (BIPMed, n.d.).	Birth location in Brazil
China Kadoorie Biobank (CKB)	China	The over half a million participants were recruited from 10 geographically defined and diverse regions of China (CKB, n.d.).	None

continued

TABLE C-1 Continued

Name	Country/ Region	Short Description	Population Descriptors Used
deCODE genetics	Iceland	This database is made up of genotypic and medical information for more than 160,000 participants which makes up over half of the adult population in Iceland. These data are used in gene discovery work (deCODE, 2016).	Geographic location in Iceland
Estonian Biobank	Estonia	Population-based biobank that has a cohort of over 200,000 individuals which makes up about 20% of the adult population in Estonia. The current cohort is reflective of the age, sex, and geographical distribution of adults in Estonia: Estonians represent 83%, Russians 14%, and other nationalities 3% (UT, 2021).	Place of birth, place(s) of living, nationality
Health and Aging in Africa: A Longitudinal Study of an INDEPTH Community in South Africa (HAALSI)	South Africa	Community-based cohort of 5,059 men and women who are 40 or older. The aim of the study is to identify characteristics of the aging process in rural South Africa (HAALSI, 2022).	Country of origin and languages spoken
Korea Biobank Project (KBP)	South Korea	The purpose of KBP is to collect and manage human bioresources for future use in research. In 2018, the biobank was made up of 852,769 participants (KBP, n.d.).	None
Malaysia Cohort Study	Malaysia	Aims to recruit 100,000 individuals aged 35–70 years to identify risk factors, gene–environment interactions, and biomarkers for cancer and other diseases (Jamal et al., 2015).	Ethnicity—Malay, Chinese, Indian, Other; Locality—urban or rural

TABLE C-1 Continued

Name	Country/Region	Short Description	Population Descriptors Used
Mexican Biobank (MXB)	Mexico	To date, they have genotyped 6,057 Mexican individuals who are linked with their demographic and medical data. The individuals were recruited from all 32 states with specific efforts made to include those who speak an Indigenous language (Sohail et al., 2022).	Geography and genetic ancestry
Prospective Epidemiological Research Studies in Iran (PERSIAN Cohort Study)	Iran	Aims to recruit 180,000 individuals aged 35–70 years from 18 regions in Iran. The study is designed to be ethnically representative and recruit across diverse geographies of the country (Poustchi et al., 2018).	Ethnicity
Qatar Biobank (QBB)	Qatar	The population cohort aims to recruit 60,000 participants. The goal of the biobank is to collect information to study how lifestyle, environment, and genes affect health locally in Qatar (Fthenou et al., 2019).	Ethnicity—Qataris, long-term residents who are members of Arab groups other than Qatari, and long-term residents of non-Arab groups. Members of Arab group other than Qatari include Algerian, Bahraini, Egyptian, Emirian, Iraqi, Jordanian, Kuwaiti, Lebanese, Mauritanian, Moroccan, Omani, Palestinian, Saudi Arabian, Somali, Sudanese, Syrian, Tunisian, Emirati, and Yemeni. Non-Arab groups include: American, Armenian, Bangladeshi, Canadian, Cypriot, Ethiopian, Indian, Iranian, Japanese, Dutch, Pakistani, Filipino, Tajikistani, and British (Al Thani et al., 2019).

continued

TABLE C-1 Continued

Name	Country/Region	Short Description	Population Descriptors Used
Singapore National Precision Medicine Program	Singapore	Three-phase program to implement precision health. Phase I collected 10,000 genomes for a reference database, phase II aims to collect 100,000 genomes of healthy individuals and 50,000 from people with specific diseases, and phase III will implement precision medicine (PRECISE, 2022).	Self-reported ethnicity, inferred ethnicity, and inferred ancestry based on genotyping
Taiwan Biobank	Taiwan	The aim of the biobank is to improve medical care. The biobank was established in 2012 and has recruited over 176,000 individuals with a goal of 200,000 participants (Wei et al., 2021).	Ancestry—Han Chinese including Taiwanese Minnan, Taiwanese Hakka, and ancestries across China: East China, South Central China, North and Northeast China, and Southwest China and other East Asian groups
National Laboratory for the Genetics of Israeli Populations	Israel	The laboratory is meant to be a national repository for DNA samples and human cell lines that are representative of the variation in Israel and several Middle Eastern populations (Mcgonigle, 2021).	Self-identified ethnicity—Palestinian, Druze, Bedouin, and Jewish. Jewish is broken down further into the following subcategories: Ashkenazi (central European ancestry), Ethiopian, Georgian, Iranian, Iraqi, Kuchin (India), Libyan, Moroccan, Sephardi (Turkey and Bulgaria), Tunisian, Yemenite
UK Biobank	United Kingdom	Genetic and health information of over half a million participants in the UK (Fry et al., 2017).	Self-reported ethnicity which includes white (white British, white Irish, and other white background), black or black British (Caribbean, African, or other black background), Mixed (white and black Caribbean, white and black African, white and Asian, and other mixed ethnic background), Indian, Pakistani, Bangladeshi, Chinese, other Asian, other ethnic group (Fry et al., 2017).

REFERENCES

Al Thani, A., E. Fthenou, S. Paparrodopoulos, A. Al Marri, Z. Shi, F. Qafoud, and N. Afifi. 2019. Qatar Biobank cohort study: Study design and first results. *American Journal of Epidemiology* 188(8):1420-1433.

BBJ (Biobank Japan). 2021. *Biobank Japan*. https://biobankjp.org/en/index.html (accessed October 24, 2022).

BIPMed (Brazilian Initiative on Precision Medicine). n.d. *About BIPMed*. https://bipmed.org/about.html (accessed October 24, 2022).

CKB (China Kadoorie Biobank). n.d. *Aims and rationale*. https://www.ckbiobank.org/about-us/aims-and-rationale (accessed October 25, 2022).

deCODE (deCODE Genetics). 2016. *Science*. https://www.decode.com/research/ (accessed October 25, 2022).

Fry, A., T. J. Littlejohns, C. Sudlow, N. Doherty, L. Adamska, T. Sprosen, R. Collins, and N. E. Allen. 2017. Comparison of sociodemographic and health-related characteristics of UK biobank participants with those of the general population. *American Journal of Epidemiology* 186(9):1026-1034.

Fthenou, E., A. Al Thani, A. Al Marri, and N. Afifi. 2019. Qatar Biobank: A paradigm of translating biobank science into evidence-based health care interventions. *Biopreservation and Biobanking* 17(6):491-493.

HAALSI (Health and Aging in Africa: A Longitudinal Study of an INDEPTH Community in South Africa). 2022. *About HAALSI*. https://haalsi.org/about (accessed October 24, 2022).

Jamal, R., S. Z. Syed Zakaria, M. A. Kamaruddin, N. Abd Jalal, N. Ismail, N. Mohd Kamil, N. Abdullah, N. Baharudin, N. H. Hussin, H. Othman, and N. M. Mahadi. 2015. Cohort profile: The Malaysian cohort (TMC) project: A prospective study of non-communicable diseases in a multi-ethnic population. *International Journal of Epidemiology* 44(2):423-431.

KBP (Korea Biobank Project). n.d. *Policy and services*. https://www.kdca.go.kr/contents.es?mid=a30326000000 (accessed October 25, 2022).

Mcgonigle, I. 2021. National biobanking in Qatar and Israel: Tracing how global scientific institutions mediate local ethnic identities. *Science, Technology and Society* 26(1):146-165.

Poustchi, H., S. Eghtesad, F. Kamangar, A. Etemadi, A. A. Keshtkar, A. Hekmatdoost, Z. Mohammadi, Z. Mahmoudi, A. Shayanrad, F. Roozafzai, M. Sheikh, A. Jalaeikhoo, M. H. Somi, F. Mansour-Ghanaei, F. Najafi, E. Bahramali, A. Mehrparvar, A. Ansari-Moghaddam, A. A. Enayati, A. Esmaeili Nadimi, A. Rezaianzadeh, N. Saki, F. Alipour, R. Kelishadi, A. Rahimi-Movaghar, N. Aminisani, P. Boffetta, and R. Malekzadeh. 2018. Prospective epidemiological research studies in Iran (the PERSIAN Cohort Study): Rationale, objectives, and design. *American Journal of Epidemiology* 187(4):647-655.

PRECISE (Singapore National Precision Medicine Program). 2022. *About us*. https://www.npm.sg/about-us/our story/ (accessed October 25, 2022).

Sohail, M., A. Y. Chong, C. D. Quinto-Cortes, M. J. Palma-Martínez, A. Ragsdale, S. G. Medina-Muñoz, C. Barberena-Jonas, G. Delgado-Sánchez, L. P. Cruz-Hervert, L. Ferreyra-Reyes, E. Ferreira-Guerrero, N. Mongua-Rodríguez, A. Jimenez-Kaufmann, H. Moreno-Macías, C. A. Aguilar-Salinas, K. Auckland, A. Cortés, V. Acuña-Alonzo, A. G. Ioannidis, C. R. Gignoux, G. L. Wojcik, S. L. Fernández-Valverde, A. V. S. Hill, M. T. Tusié-Luna, A. J. Mentzer, J. Novembre, L. García-García, and A. Moreno-Estrada. 2022. Nationwide genomic biobank in Mexico unravels demographic history and complex trait architecture from 6,057 individuals. *bioRxiv* 2022.07.11.499652.

UT (University of Tartu). 2021. *Estonian biobank*. https://genomics.ut.ee/en/content/estonian-biobank (accessed October 25, 2022).

Wei, C.-Y., J.-H. Yang, E.-C. Yeh, M.-F. Tsai, H.-J. Kao, C.-Z. Lo, L.-P. Chang, W.-J. Lin, F.-J. Hsieh, S. Belsare, A. Bhaskar, M.-W. Su, T.-C. Lee, Y.-L. Lin, F.-T. Liu, C.-Y. Shen, L.-H. Li, C.-H. Chen, J. D. Wall, J.-Y. Wu, and P.-Y. Kwok. 2021. Genetic profiles of 103,106 individuals in the Taiwan biobank provide insights into the health and history of Han Chinese. *Genomic Medicine* 6(1):10.

D

Decision Tree for the Use of Population Descriptors in Genomics Research

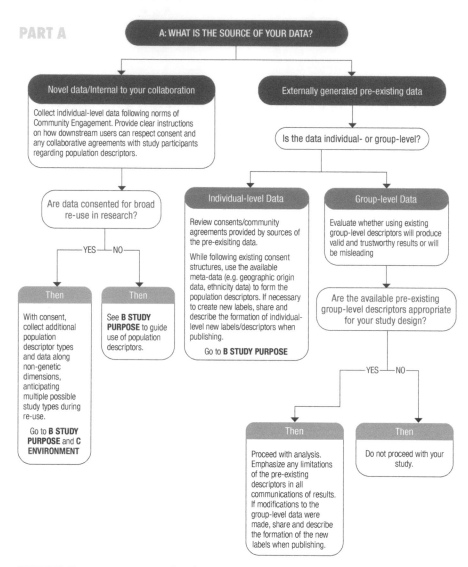

FIGURE D-1 Decision tree for the use of population descriptors in genomics research. The decision tree follows on the next several pages.

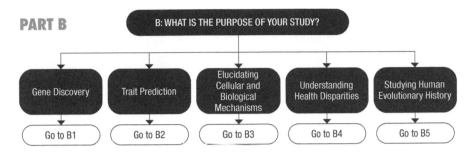

FIGURE D-1 Continued

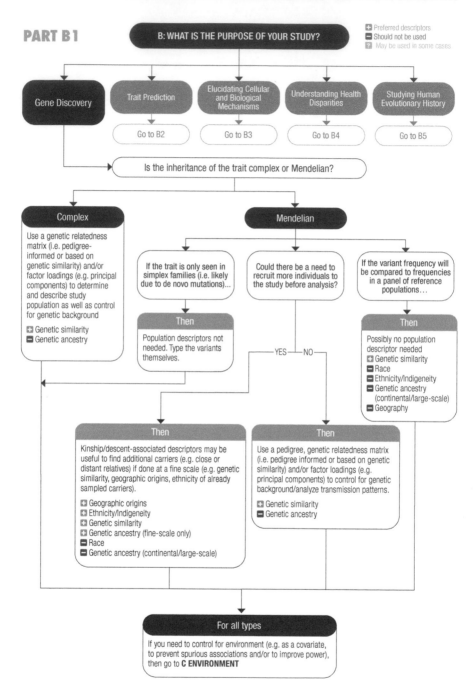

FIGURE D-1 Continued

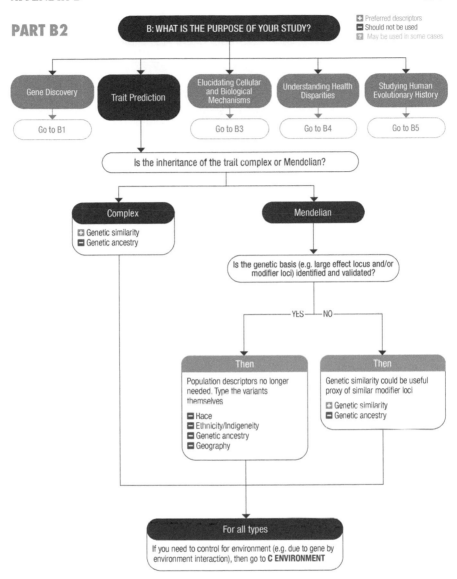

FIGURE D-1 Continued

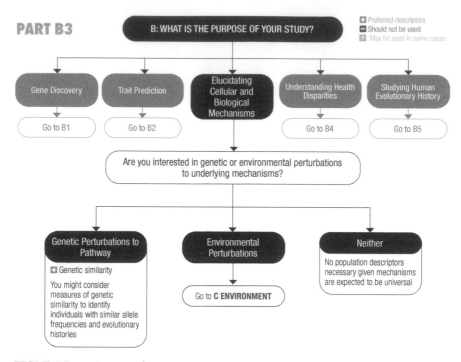

FIGURE D-1 Continued

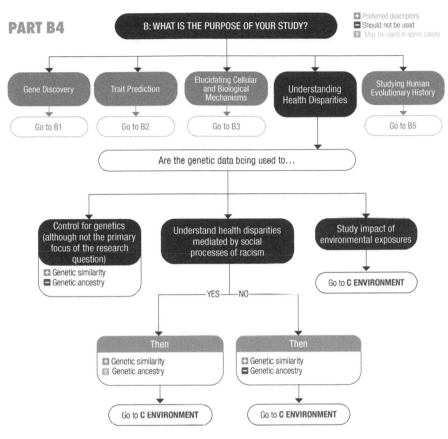

FIGURE D-1 Continued

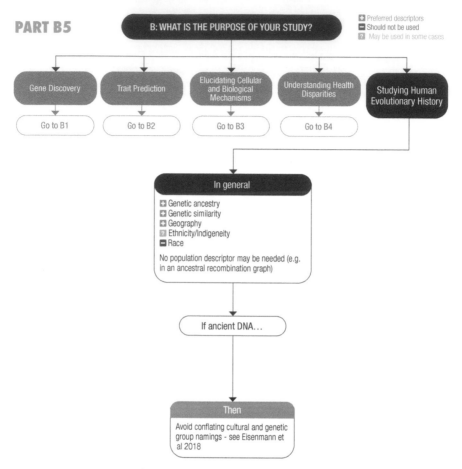

FIGURE D-1 Continued

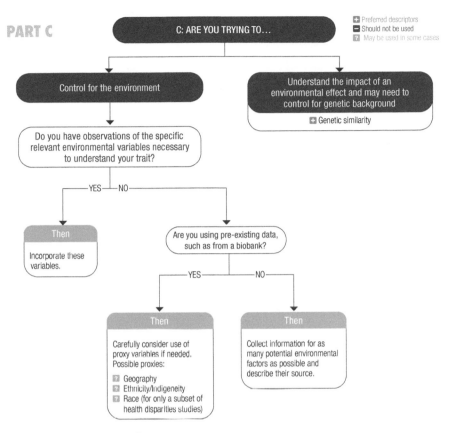

FIGURE D-1 Continued

E

Committee and Staff Biosketches

COMMITTEE MEMBER BIOSKETCHES

Aravinda Chakravarti, Ph.D. (*Cochair*), is the director of the Center for Human Genetics & Genomics, and the Muriel G. & George W. Singer Professor of Neuroscience & Physiology and professor of medicine at the New York University Grossman School of Medicine. He has served on the faculty at the University of Pittsburgh (1980–1993), Case Western Reserve University (1994–2000), and Johns Hopkins University (2000–2018). He is one of the founding Editors-in-Chief of *Genome Research* and *Annual Review of Genomics and Human Genetics* and has been or is on the advisory boards of numerous national and international institutes, charities, academic societies, the National Institutes of Health, and biotechnology companies. He has been a key participant in many genome projects, and now works on genome-scale analysis of the molecular basis of human disease. He was the 2008 President of the American Society of Human Genetics and has been elected to the U.S. National Academy of Sciences, the U.S. National Academy of Medicine, the Indian National Academy of Science, and the Indian Academy of Sciences. He was awarded the 2013 William Allan Award by the American Society of Human Genetics and the 2018 Chen Award by the Human Genome Organization. Dr. Chakravarti received his Ph.D. in human genetics in 1979.

Charmaine Royal, Ph.D. (*Cochair*), is the Robert O. Keohane Professor of African & African American Studies, Biology, Global Health, and Family Medicine & Community Health at Duke University. She directs the Duke

Center on Genomics, Race, Identity, Difference and the Duke Center for Truth, Racial Healing & Transformation. She held previous faculty appointments at Howard University. Throughout her career, Dr. Royal has focused on ethical, social, scientific, and clinical implications of human genetics and genomics, particularly issues at the intersection of genetics and "race." She serves on numerous national and international advisory boards and committees for government agencies, professional organizations, not-for-profit entities, and corporations, including the Board of Directors for the American Society of Human Genetics, the Independent Expert Committee for the Human Heredity and Health in Africa (H3Africa) Initiative, and the Ethics Advisory Board for Illumina, Inc. In 2013 and 2015 Dr. Royal served as a chairperson of the planning committee for two consensus roundtable meetings convened by the American Society of Human Genetics charged with developing guidelines for genetic ancestry inference. Dr. Royal obtained a bachelor's degree in microbiology, master's degree in genetic counseling, and doctorate in human genetics from Howard University. She completed postgraduate training in ethical, legal, and social implications (ELSI) research and bioethics at the National Human Genome Research Institute of the National Institutes of Health, and in epidemiology and behavioral medicine at Howard University Cancer Center. She was a member of the National Academies committees that produced *Toward Precision Medicine: Building a Knowledge Network for Biomedical Research and a New Taxonomy of Disease* and *Addressing Sickle Cell Disease: A Strategic Plan and Blueprint for Action.*

Katrina Armstrong, M.D., leads Columbia University's medical campus as the Executive Vice President for Health and Biomedical Sciences. She is Chief Executive Officer of the Columbia University Irving Medical Center and Dean of the Faculties of Health Sciences and Medicine, which includes Columbia's dental, medical, nursing, and public health schools. She is an internationally recognized investigator in medical decision making, quality of care, and cancer prevention and outcomes, an award-winning teacher, and a practicing primary care physician. She has served on multiple advisory panels for academic and federal organizations and has been elected to the National Academy of Medicine, the American Academy of Arts and Sciences, the Association of American Physicians, and the American Society for Clinical Investigation. Before joining Columbia, Dr. Armstrong was the Jackson Professor of Clinical Medicine at Harvard Medical School, Chair of the Department of Medicine, Physician-in-Chief of Massachusetts General Hospital, and Professor of Epidemiology at the Harvard T. H. Chan School of Public Health. Before joining Harvard, she was Chief of the Division of General Internal Medicine, Associate Director of the Abramson Cancer Center, and Codirector of the Robert Wood Johnson Clinical Scholars Program at the University of Pennsylvania. She is a graduate of Yale University

(B.A. degree in architecture), Johns Hopkins (M.D. degree), and the University of Pennsylvania (M.S. degree in clinical epidemiology). She completed her residency training in internal medicine at Johns Hopkins.

Michael Bamshad, M.D., is professor and chief of the Division of Genetic Medicine in the Department of Pediatrics at the University of Washington and Seattle Children's Hospital, and holds the Allan and Phyllis Treuer Endowed Chair in Genetics and Development. Dr. Bamshad is Editor-in-Chief of *Human Genetics and Genomics Advances*, published by the American Society of Human Genetics, and chair of the Scientific Advisory Board of GeneDx. His research focuses on understanding the effect of population structure and natural selection on human genetic variation; developing innovative ways to discover genetic variants underlying monogenic disorders, modifiers of monogenic traits, and complex traits; and testing novel ways to translate genomic advances into the practice of precision genetic medicine. He and his colleagues pioneered the use of exome and genome sequencing for discovery of genes underlying Mendelian conditions and has contributed to the identification of hundreds of genes for Mendelian disorders. He has also been a leader in understanding the relationship between genetic ancestry and notions of race, developing innovative ways to openly share phenotypic information and genetic data (e.g., MyGene2) and building platforms for self-guided return of genetic testing results (e.g., My46) from exome and whole genome sequencing in both research and clinical settings. He has published more than 300 scientific manuscripts as well as papers in periodicals such as *Scientific American* and coauthors a popular textbook titled *Medical Genetics*. In 2013 and 2015 Dr. Bamshad served as a chairperson of the planning committee for two consensus roundtable meetings convened by the American Society of Human Genetics charged with developing guidelines for genetic ancestry inference. He received his B.S. and M.D. at the University of Missouri in Kansas City and his M.A. at the University of Kansas.

Luisa N. Borrell, D.D.S., Ph.D., is a distinguished professor in the Department of Epidemiology and Biostatistics, City University of New York Graduate School of Public Health and Health Policy (CUNY SPH) in New York. She is a social epidemiologist with a research interest in the role of race/ethnicity, socioeconomic position, and neighborhood effects as social determinants of health. Her work on Hispanics'/Latinos' racial identity brings attention to the need for disaggregated analyses by race as Hispanics/Latinos are a heterogeneous group with a mix of European, Native American, and African ancestry. She also has expertise in research methods and analyses of large and spatially linked data sets. Dr. Borrell is a Fellow of the New York Academy of Medicine. She has a doctor in dental surgery and a master in public health from Columbia University, New York, as well as a doctorate in epidemiological science from the University of Michigan, Ann Arbor.

Katrina Claw, Ph.D., is an assistant professor in the Department of Biomedical Informatics in the School of Medicine at the University of Colorado Anschutz Medical Campus. Her research focuses broadly on personalizing medicine, using genetic information and biomarkers for tailored treatment, in relation to pharmacogenomics, as well as understanding the cultural, ethical, legal, and social implications of genomic research with populations historically underrepresented in health research. Her current research includes studying cytochrome P450 genetic variation in Indigenous communities (e.g., American Indian and Alaska Native peoples). Her other projects include exploring the perspectives of tribal members on genetic research with tribes and developing guidelines and policies in partnership with tribes. All of her projects strive to use community-based participatory research approaches and include cultural and Indigenous knowledge. She was awarded the Genomic Innovator Award from the National Human Genome Research Institute in 2020 for her work on pharmacogenomics approaches to drug metabolism in American Indian/Alaska Native people. She received her B.S. and B.A. from Arizona State University and her Ph.D. from the University of Washington.

Clarence C. Gravlee, Ph.D., is an associate professor in the Department of Anthropology at the University of Florida, where he is also affiliated with the Center for Latin American Studies, the African American Studies Program, and the Genetics Institute. His research examines the genetic and environmental contributors to hypertension in the African diaspora, with an emphasis on the biological consequences of systemic racism. His work, with collaborators, integrates methods and theory from the social and biological sciences, including ethnography, social network analysis, human biology, and genetics. Gravlee completed a B.A., M.A., and Ph.D. in anthropology at the University of Florida, a Fulbright graduate fellowship at the Universität zu Köln (Cologne, Germany), and postdoctoral training in community-based participatory research as a W.K. Kellogg Community Health Scholar at the University of Michigan School of Public Health.

Mark D. Hayward, Ph.D., is a professor of sociology and Centennial Commission Professor in the Liberal Arts at the University of Texas at Austin. Hayward is a health demographer. Building on a long-standing interest in the developmental origins of adult health, his current work incorporates biosocial lenses (e.g., pathophysiological pathways and genetic risk) to better understand how social exposures from childhood through adulthood influence racial/ethnic disparities in dementia risk. Hayward is a recipient of the Matilda White Riley Award from the National Institutes of Health (NIH) for his contributions to behavioral and social scientific knowledge relevant to the mission of NIH. He has served on numerous major foundations (Robert Wood Johnson and Pew) and major federal agencies (e.g., the National Institutes of Health and the National Center for Health Statistics). Hayward is the current editor of his field's major journal, *Demography*, and President-elect of the Interdisciplinary Association of Population Health Science. He received his Ph.D. from Indiana University and his B.A. from Washington State University. He has served on scientific advisory boards at the National Academies of Sciences, Engineering, and Medicine including the Committee on Population and a Decadal Survey of Behavioral and Social Science Research on Alzheimer's Disease and Alzheimer's Disease-Related Dementias.

Rick Kittles, Ph.D., is Senior Vice President for Research at Morehouse School of Medicine. Dr. Kittles was previously professor and founding director of the Division of Health Equities within the Department of Population Sciences at the City of Hope (COH) and associate director of Health Equities of COH Comprehensive Cancer Center. Dr. Kittles is also Cofounder and Scientific Director of African Ancestry, Inc., and is well known for his research of prostate cancer and health disparities among African Americans, having published more than 260 research articles. Dr. Kittles serves on many national and international steering committees and advisory boards. He served as a member of the Board of Scientific Counselors for the National Human Genome Research Institute (NIH) and is Past Council Chair of the Minorities in Cancer Research of the American Association for Cancer Research. Dr. Kittles' research has focused on understanding the complex issues surrounding race, genetic ancestry, and health disparities. He has been at the forefront of the development of genetic markers for ancestry and how genetic ancestry can be used in genetics studies on disease risk and outcomes, showing the effect of genetic variation across populations. He received a Ph.D. in biological sciences from George Washington University in 1998.

Sandra Soo-Jin Lee, Ph.D., is a professor of medical humanities and ethics and chief of the Division of Ethics at Columbia University. Trained as a medical anthropologist, Dr. Lee leads interdisciplinary bioethics research on race, ancestry and equity in genomics, precision medicine, and artificial intelligence, and publishes in the genomics, medical, bioethics, and social science literatures. Dr. Lee has investigated racial categorization in human genetics for over two decades and coedited *Revisiting Race in a Genomic Age* (2008). Her current NIH-funded projects include the Ethics of

Inclusion: Diversity in Precision Medicine Research. Dr. Lee is codirector of the Center for ELSI Resources and Analysis and the ELSI Congress. She is president of the Association of Bioethics Program Directors and a Hastings Center Fellow. Dr. Lee serves on the U.S. Health and Human Services Secretary's Advisory Committee on Human Research Protections, the Scientific Advisory Boards of the Kaiser Permanente National Research Biobank and the Human Pangenome Reference Consortium, and the editorial boards of the *American Journal of Bioethics* and *Narrative Inquiry in Bioethics*. Dr. Lee received her doctorate from the University of California, Berkeley/UCSF joint program in medical anthropology and her undergraduate degree in human biology from Stanford University.

Andrés Moreno-Estrada, Ph.D., M.D., is the principal investigator of the Human Evolutionary and Population Genomics Laboratory at the Advanced Genomics Unit (UGA-CINVESTAV), in Irapuato, Mexico. Previously, he was research associate of the Genetics Department at Stanford University until 2014. He is a Mexican population geneticist interested in human genetic diversity and its implications in population history and medical genomics. His work integrates genomics, evolution, and precision medicine in projects involving large collections of understudied populations, in particular from the Americas and the Pacific. He authored the most detailed work so far of the genetic structure of the Mexican population, including the first genomic characterization of 20 diverse indigenous groups throughout Mexico, as well as fine-scale studies in the Caribbean region, South America, and Polynesia. He is leading the Human Cell Map of Latin American Diversity to increase the representation of diverse ancestry networks for the Human Cell Atlas project. For his work in Latin America he was awarded the George Rosenkranz Prize for Health Care Research in Developing Countries in 2012. He received his M.D. from University of Guadalajara in 2002 and Ph.D. in evolutionary genetics from Pompeu Fabra University in 2009. Dr. Moreno was a postdoctoral fellow until 2012 with Professor Carlos Bustamante at Cornell University and Stanford University School of Medicine.

Ann Morning, Ph.D., is the James Weldon Johnson Professor of Sociology at New York University. Trained in demography, her research focuses on race, ethnicity, and the sociology of science, especially as they pertain to census classification worldwide and to individuals' concepts of difference. She is the author of *The Nature of Race: How Scientists Think and Teach about Human Difference* (University of California Press 2011), and coauthor of *An Ugly Word: Rethinking Race in Italy and the United States* (with Marcello Maneri, Russell Sage Foundation, 2022). Morning was a 2008–2009 Fulbright research fellow at the University of Milan-Bicocca and a 2014–2015 Visiting Scholar at the Russell Sage Foundation. She was a member of the U.S. Census Bureau's National Advisory Committee on Racial, Ethnic and Other Populations from 2013 to 2019 and has consulted on racial statistics for the European Commission, the United Nations, Elsevier, and the World Bank. Morning holds her B.A. in economics and political science from Yale University, a master's of international affairs from Columbia University, and her Ph.D. in sociology from Princeton University.

John P. Novembre, Ph.D., is a professor at the University of Chicago in the Departments of Human Genetics and Ecology & Evolution. His research has developed computational methods to answer a diverse range of questions regarding genetic diversity. His work has especially had an impact on the understanding and analysis of geographic patterns in human genetic variation. He has been awarded as a MacArthur Fellow, Searle Scholar, and Sloan Research Fellow, and his research is supported by the National Institutes of Health. Dr. Novembre has authored more than 50 peer-reviewed publications in leading journals, including *Nature, Science, Nature Genetics,* and the *American Journal of Human Genetics.* He also serves as an academic editor for the journal *Genetics,* and previously served on the Scientific Advisory Board for AncestryDNA. He received his B.A. from the Colorado College and his Ph.D. from the University of California-Berkeley.

Molly Przeworski, Ph.D., is a professor of biological sciences at Columbia University. Before moving to Columbia University, she was a faculty member at the University of Chicago as well as at Brown University and the Max Planck Institute for Evolutionary Anthropology in Germany. Her research aims to understand the genetic basis and evolutionary history of heritable differences among individuals; recent work focuses in part on genomic trait prediction in humans and implications. She is the recipient of the Rosalind Franklin Award from the Genetics Society of America, a Sloan Research Fellowship, and the Howard Hughes Medical Institute Early Career Scientist Award, and she is a member of the American Academy of Arts and Sciences and the National Academy of Sciences. She received a B.A. in mathematics from Princeton University and a Ph.D. from the Committee on Evolutionary Biology at the University of Chicago, then conducted postdoctoral research in the Mathematical Genetics group of the University of Oxford in the United Kingdom.

Dorothy E. Roberts, J.D., is the George A. Weiss University Professor of Law & Sociology at University of Pennsylvania, with joint appointments in the Departments of Africana Studies and Sociology and the Law School, where she is the inaugural Raymond Pace and Sadie Tanner Mossell Alexander Professor of Civil Rights. She is also Founding Director of the Penn

Program on Race, Science & Society. Author of *Fatal Invention: How Science, Politics, and Big Business Re-create Race in the Twenty-First Century*, Roberts is an expert on structural racism in U.S. science and medicine and the use of race as a variable in scientific research. Her research has been supported by the American Council of Learned Societies, National Science Foundation, Robert Wood Johnson Foundation, Fulbright Program, Harvard Program on Ethics & the Professions, and Stanford Center for the Comparative Studies in Race & Ethnicity. Recent honors include 2022 election to the American Academy of Arts and Sciences, 2019 election as a College of Physicians of Philadelphia Fellow, 2017 election to the National Academy of Medicine, 2016 Society of Family Planning Lifetime Achievement Award, 2015 American Psychiatric Association Solomon Carter Fuller Award, and 2011 election as a Hastings Center Fellow. Professor Roberts serves on the advisory board for the Center for Genetics and Society. She received her J.D. from Harvard Law School and her B.A., magna cum laude, Phi Beta Kappa, from Yale College.

Sarah A. Tishkoff, Ph.D., is the David and Lyn Silfen University Professor in Genetics and Biology at the University of Pennsylvania, holding appointments in the School of Medicine and the School of Arts and Sciences. She is also the director of the Penn Center for Global Genomics & Health Equity. Dr. Tishkoff studies genomic and phenotypic variation in ethnically diverse Africans, using field work, laboratory research, and computational methods to examine African population history, the genetic basis of anthropometric, cardiovascular, and immune-related traits, and how humans have adapted to diverse environments and diets. Dr. Tishkoff is a member of the National Academy of Sciences (NAS), the American Academy of Arts and Sciences, and the National Academy of Medicine. She is a recipient of an NIH Pioneer Award, a David and Lucile Packard Career Award, a Burroughs/Wellcome Fund Career Award, the ASHG Curt Stern Award, and a Penn Integrates Knowledge (PIK) endowed chair. She is on the NAS Board of Global Health and the Scientific Advisory Board for the Packard Fellowships in Science and Engineering, and is on the editorial boards at *Cell*, *PLoS Genetics*, and *G3* (*Genes, Genomes, and Genetics*). She received her Ph.D. in genetics and M.Phil. in human genetics from Yale University and her B.S. in anthropology and genetics from University of California-Berkeley.

Genevieve L. Wojcik, Ph.D., is an assistant professor of epidemiology at the Johns Hopkins Bloomberg School of Public Health in Baltimore, Maryland. As a statistical geneticist and genetic epidemiologist, her research focuses on method development for diverse populations, specifically understanding the role of genetic ancestry and environment in genetic risk in admixed populations. Dr. Wojcik integrates epidemiology, sociology, and population genetics to better understand existing health disparities in minority populations, as well as underserved populations globally. In 2021, she was the recipient of one of NHGRI's Genomic Innovator Awards (R35) to do this work. She is a long-standing member of multiple NHGRI consortia focused on diverse populations, such as the Population Architecture using Genomics and Epidemiology (PAGE) Study, which was formed by NHGRI over a decade ago to address the lack of genetics research in non-European ancestry populations, and the PRIMED consortium, which began in 2022 to better conduct research around polygenic risk scores in diverse populations. Dr. Wojcik previously served as a consultant with Illumina, Inc. Prior to her faculty appointment, Dr. Wojcik was a postdoctoral research scholar at Stanford University in the Departments of Genetics and Biomedical Data Science. She received her Ph.D. in epidemiology and M.H.S. in human genetics/genetic epidemiology from the Johns Hopkins Bloomberg School of Public Health and her B.A. in biology from Cornell University.

STAFF BIOSKETCHES

Sarah H. Beachy, Ph.D. (*Study Director*), is a senior program officer with the National Academies of Sciences, Engineering, and Medicine. In this capacity, Dr. Beachy serves as Director of the Roundtable on Genomics and Precision Health and the Forum on Regenerative Medicine, in addition to leading other projects. In these roles, she has facilitated impactful activities on topics such as Improving Diversity of the Genomics Workforce, Understanding Disparities in Access to Genomic Medicine, Changing the Culture of Data Sharing and Management, and An Examination of Emerging Bioethical Issues in Biomedical Research, among others. In 2022, Sarah was awarded a National Academy of Medicine Cecil Award for Individual Excellence for her contributions to the National Academies. Prior to her time at the National Academies, Dr. Beachy completed an AAAS Science and Technology Policy Fellowship in diplomacy at the U.S. Department of State, working closely with the Office of the Science and Technology Adviser to the Secretary. She was selected as a Mirzayan Science and Technology Policy Fellow at the National Academies in 2011. Prior to moving into science policy, Dr. Beachy was a postdoctoral fellow in the Genetics Branch at the National Cancer Institute, where she generated and characterized transgenic mouse models of leukemia and lymphoma. She earned her Ph.D. in biophysics from the Roswell Park Cancer Institute Graduate Division at the University at Buffalo.

Samantha N. Schumm, Ph.D., is an associate program officer with the Board on Health Sciences Policy at the National Academies of Sciences, Engineering, and Medicine. Prior to joining the National Academies, she studied mild traumatic brain injury at the University of Pennsylvania, using a variety of neuroscience techniques. Dr. Schumm developed a novel computational network model of the hippocampus and analyzed emergent complex behaviors of neuronal networks. Her other interests include writing and promoting effective, inclusive mentorship in the sciences. Dr. Schumm holds a Ph.D. in bioengineering from the University of Pennsylvania and a B.S. in biomedical engineering from Yale University.

Leah Cairns, Ph.D. (*Study Codirector, until October 2022*), is a program officer in the Board on Health Sciences Policy. Her primary interests include health policy and biomedical research. Prior to joining the National Academies, she served as an AAAS Science and Technology Policy Fellow working as legislative staff for a member of Congress focusing on health policy and appropriations. Dr. Cairns also previously served as a Christine Mirzayan Science & Technology Policy Fellow at the National Academies in the Policy and Global Affairs Division. Dr. Cairns received her Ph.D. in biophysics from the Johns Hopkins University School of Medicine and a B.A. in biochemistry and molecular biology from Hamilton College.

Kathryn Asalone, Ph.D., is an associate program officer in the Board on Health Sciences Policy at the National Academies of Sciences, Engineering, and Medicine. Her primary interests include genomics research, science communication, and diversity, equity, inclusion, and justice issues. Prior to her time at the National Academies, she studied the germline restricted chromosome in zebra finch using computational genomics methods. Dr. Asalone received her Ph.D. in behavior, cognition, and neuroscience and M.A. in psychology from American University and a B.S. in zoology from the University of Maine.

Meredith Hackmann is an associate program officer on the Board on Health Sciences Policy at the National Academies of Sciences, Engineering, and Medicine. She joined the National Academies in 2014 and has facilitated public workshops, action collaboratives, and working groups with the Roundtable on Genomics and Precision Health and the Forum on Regenerative Medicine. She recently supported a consensus study on A Fairer and More Equitable, Cost-Effective, and Transparent System of Donor Organ Procurement, Allocation, and Distribution. She has provided background research and writing support for proceedings and consensus studies within the Board on Health Sciences Policy on topics such as bioethics, implementing genomic screening programs, digital health, and consumer genomics. Prior to joining the Academies, she was an intern with the U.S. House of Representatives. She earned a bachelor's degree in international studies from the University of Missouri and is currently pursuing a master's degree in public affairs.

Lydia Teferra is a research assistant with the Board on Health Sciences at the National Academies of Sciences, Engineering, and Medicine, serving as a staff member with the Roundtable on Genomics and Precision Health and the Forum on Regenerative Medicine. She graduated from Northwestern University in 2020 with a B.A. in psychology and global health and has been working at the National Academies for more than a year. Prior to her time at the National Academies, Ms. Teferra interned and volunteered for local nonprofit organizations addressing a number of public health issues. She hopes to pursue a master's degree in public health in the near future.

Aparna Cheran is a senior program assistant with the Board on Health Sciences Policy at the National Academies of Sciences, Engineering, and Medicine. She graduated from Virginia Polytechnic Institute and State University in 2020 with a B.S. in microbiology, and a B.A. in religion and culture. She is currently pursuing a master's in health administration from George Mason University, and hopes to establish a career in global health in the future.

Michael Zierler, Ph.D., is the founder and co-owner of RedOx Scientific Editing, a small shop that provides developmental editing and related editorial and writing services. He has an undergraduate degree in biology from Brown University and a Ph.D. in biology from Johns Hopkins University, where he worked on the regulation of gene expression in eukaryotes, stockpiling of DNA polymerases during embryogenesis, and intramolecular movements in hemoglobin studied using hydrogen exchange. Prior to graduate school, he spent a summer studying the behavior of lemon sharks off the Florida Keys and worked for a cardiothoracic surgeon at the West Roxbury Veterans Affairs Medical Center, doing research in the laboratory and the operating room on monitoring and improving the physiology of the heart during open heart surgery using mass spectrometry and a miniaturized pH electrode. After graduate school, he completed a postdoctoral position at the State University of New York, Stony Brook, helping to identify the molecular components of the Salmonella injectisome, a bacterial invasion system. He has taught biological sciences at the high school and college levels. He has also served as the deputy mayor and the chair of the planning board in his hometown of New Paltz, New York.

Andrew M. Pope, Ph.D. (*until July 2022*), was the director of the Board on Health Sciences Policy until retiring in the summer of 2022. He has a Ph.D. in physiology and biochemistry from the University of Maryland and has been a member of the National Academies of Sciences, Engineering, and

Medicine staff since 1982, and of the Health and Medicine Division staff since 1989. His primary interests are science policy, biomedical ethics, and environmental and occupational influences on human health. During his tenure at the Academies, Dr. Pope has directed numerous studies on topics that range from injury control, disability prevention, and biologic markers to the protection of human research participants, National Institutes of Health priority-setting processes, organ procurement and transplantation policy, and the role of science and technology in countering terrorism. Since 1998, Dr. Pope has served as Director of the Board on Health Sciences Policy, which oversees and guides a program of activities that is intended to encourage and sustain the continuous vigor of the basic biomedical and clinical research enterprises needed to ensure and improve the health and resilience of the public. Ongoing activities include Forums on Neuroscience, Genomics, Drug Discovery and Development, and Medical and Public Health Preparedness for Catastrophic Events. Dr. Pope is the recipient of the Health and Medicine Division's Cecil Award and the National Academy of Sciences President's Special Achievement Award.

Clare Stroud, Ph.D. *(from July 2022)*, is the senior board director for the Board on Health Sciences Policy. In this capacity, she oversees a program of activities aimed at fostering the basic biomedical and clinical research enterprises; addressing the ethical, legal, and social contexts of scientific and technologic advances related to health; and strengthening the preparedness, resilience, and sustainability of communities. Previously, she served as director of the National Academies' Forum on Neuroscience and Nervous System Disorders, which brings together leaders from government, academia, industry, and nonprofit organizations to discuss key challenges and emerging issues in neuroscience research, development of therapies for nervous system disorders, and related ethical and societal issues. She also led consensus studies and contributed to projects on topics such as pain management, medications for opioid use disorder, traumatic brain injury, preventing cognitive decline and dementia, supporting persons living with dementia and their caregivers, the health and well-being of young adults, and disaster preparedness and response. Dr. Stroud first joined the National Academies as a Christine Mirzayan Science and Technology Policy Graduate Fellow. She has also been an associate at AmericaSpeaks, a nonprofit organization that engaged citizens in decision making on important public policy issues. Dr. Stroud received her Ph.D. from the University of Maryland, College Park, with research focused on the cognitive neuroscience of language, and her bachelor's degree from Queen's University in Canada.

Malay K. Majmundar, J.D., Ph.D., directs the Committee on Population (CPOP). He is currently overseeing CPOP activities on social and economic mobility, structural racism, and the workplace and aging. He is also developing a future research portfolio for CPOP. While at the National Academies, he has worked on studies on demography, criminal justice, immigration enforcement and statistics, and the federal budget. He has a B.A. in political science from Duke University, a J.D. from Yale University, and a Ph.D. in public policy from the University of Chicago.

F

Disclosure of Unavoidable
Conflict of Interest

The conflict-of-interest policy of the National Academies of Sciences, Engineering, and Medicine (https://www.nationalacademies.org/about/institutional-policies-and-procedures/conflict-of-interest-policies-and-procedures) prohibits the appointment of an individual to a committee like the one that authored this Consensus Study Report if the individual has a conflict of interest that is relevant to the task to be performed. An exception to this prohibition is permitted only if the National Academies determine that the conflict is unavoidable and the conflict is promptly and publicly disclosed.

When the committee that authored this report was established, a determination of whether there was a conflict of interest was made for each committee member given the individual's circumstances and the task being undertaken by the committee. A determination that an individual has a conflict of interest is not an assessment of that individual's actual behavior or character or ability to act objectively despite the conflicting interest.

Dr. Rick Kittles was determined to have a conflict of interest because of his financial interests in African Ancestry, Inc., a provider of at-home genetic ancestry tests for people of African descent, which could be one way to identify people for genomic research applications. The National Academies determined that the experience and expertise of the individual was needed for the committee to accomplish the task for which it was established. The National Academies could not find another available individual with the equivalent experience and expertise who did not have a conflict of interest. Therefore, the National Academies concluded that the conflict was unavoidable and publicly disclosed it on its website (www.nationalacademies.org).